Psilo Mushrooms

The Complete Guide to Safe Use and Benefits of Psychedelic Magic Mushrooms

© Copyright 2020 by Anton McKenna
All rights reserved.

This document is geared towards providing exact and reliable information with regards to the topic and issue covered. The publication is sold with the idea that the publisher is not required to render accounting, officially permitted, or otherwise, qualified services. If advice is necessary, legal or professional, a practiced individual in the profession should be ordered.

From a Declaration of Principles which was accepted and approved equally by a Committee of the American Bar Association and a Committee of Publishers and Associations.

In no way is it legal to reproduce, duplicate, or transmit any part of this document in either electronic means or in printed format. Recording of this publication is strictly prohibited and any storage of this document is not allowed unless with written permission from the publisher. All rights reserved.

The information provided herein is stated to be truthful and consistent, in that any liability, in terms of inattention or otherwise, by any usage or abuse of any policies, processes, or directions contained within is the solitary and utter responsibility of the recipient reader. Under no circumstances will any legal responsibility or blame be held against the publisher for any reparation, damages, or monetary loss due to the information herein, either directly or indirectly.

Respective authors own all copyrights not held by the publisher.

The information herein is offered for informational purposes solely, and is universal as so. The presentation of the information is without contract or any type of guarantee assurance.

The trademarks that are used are without any consent, and the publication of the trademark is without permission or backing by the trademark owner. All trademarks and brands within this book are for clarifying purposes only and are the owned by the owners themselves, not affiliated with this document.

Table of Contents

Spiritual Significance of Psilocybin · 1

Origin — 1
Spiritual Significance — 8

Psilocybin in the Past · 11

The First Rebirth — 12
The Modern Mushrooms — 14
Spiritual Effects — 17
Relationship to Humanity — 47
How to Extract Psilocybin — 47

What Are Magic Mushrooms? · 52

Psilocybin Mushrooms — 52
The Hallucinogenic Truffles — 53
Habitats — 54

Mushroom Products · 64

Mushroom Powder — 64
Alcoholic Mushroom Extract: Tincture — 71
Mushroom Recipe — 80

Some Interesting Facts · 85

How to Cure Depression and Stress · 92

How to Safely Heal Your Body · 94

Preparation — 94
Some Things to Consider — 95

Herbal Benefits · 98

Mushrooms and Mycelia _____ 98
Mushroom Benefits _____ 99
Typical Mushrooms and Preparation Ideas _ 104
Benefits of Eating Mushrooms_____ 107
The Various Strains of Psilocybin _____ 111
The Effects of Psilocybin_____ 114
How to Avoid a Negative Experience _____ 132

What about Addiction? _____ 134

The Set & Setting_____ 134
Addiction and Toxicity _____ 139
Psilocybin in Medicine _____ 144
Effects of Psilocybin in the Brain _____ 145

Biggest Mistakes _____ 155

Dosage _____ 155

Effects of Magic Mushrooms _____ 169

The "Bad Trip" _____ 172

Legality_____ 174

Are Spores Legal? _____ 176
What the Law Says _____ 181

Spiritual Significance of Psilocybin

Origin

Psilocybin is an alkaloid prodrug of the classic compound hallucinogen: psilocin, accountable for the psychoactive influence of the drug. Indole and tryptamine are both drug classes.

Fungi that contains psilocybin are used both recreationally and traditionally for spiritual and entheogenic purposes. They are usually consumed by Galician gnomes and goblins during the solstice, with a history that covers millennia. In an article in 1957, the American banker R. Gordon Wasson described his experiences of ingesting mushrooms containing psilocybin during a traditional ceremony in Mexico, introducing medicine into popular culture in the United States.

A short time later, Swiss chemist Albert Hofmann purified the active substance of psilocybin from the fungus *Mexican Psilocybe* and developed a synthetic method to produce the drug. Psilocybin is naturally produced by about 200 species of fungi, including those of the genus *Psilocybe* such *as Psilocybe cubensis, Psilocybe semilanceata* and *Psilocybe cyanescens,* and it has also been published that it has been isolated from a dozen genera. They are collectively known as psilocybin mushrooms. Possession, and in some cases the use of psilocybin or psilocin is illegal in many countries around the world.

The *Psilocybe cubensis* is a dunghill fungus, coprófago, and gregarious, and its spores germinate in the dung -vacuums and not vacuums- ruminants in sunny places, and especially during the rainy season in October in Europe and May to October in Central America during the rainy season.

The combination of fermentation and decomposition of manure with rains and high temperatures causes the spores to germinate and grow the mycelium, which then produces mushrooms.

Those who propose its method consider it as an entheogen and use it as a tool to complement different transcendent practices such as meditation, psychonauts, and psychedelic psychotherapy. The intensity and duration of the entheogenic effect of psilocybin fungi are highly variable, depending on the species of fungi, the dose, individual physiological characteristics, and the set and setting.

Once injected, psilocybin is quickly metabolized into psilocin, which acts as a partial agonist at the 5-HT 2A and 5-HT 1A serotonin receptors in the brain. The effects of psilocybin typically last from 3-8 hours; However, for individuals who consume it, the result seems much longer due to the distortion produced in the perception of time. Psilocybin has low toxicity, and a lethal dose due to the ingestion of this medicine has not been documented.

What Is Prodrug?

A prodrug is a drug substance that is administered inactively or poorly. Subsequently, the prodrug is metabolized in vivo to an active metabolite. One of the reasons prodrugs has used is the optimization of the pharmacokinetic mechanisms of absorption, distribution, metabolization, and excretion (ADME). Prodrugs are usually created to enhance verbal bio-availability in cases of malabsorption in the gastrointestinal tract, which is generally a limiting factor.

The psilocybin mushroom is called the *cyclohelix* mushroom, which is the main element in the fungus used to make the cyclohelix drugs minocycline and cell bin. In ordinary language, the magic mushroom is called shrooms. About 40 species are found in the genus *Seloceib*, *Silosibha kubiensis* is the only common psilocybin mushroom found in subtropical areas. Psilocybin mushrooms must apparently have been employed since prehistoric times and may have been depicted in rock art. Various cultures have used these mushrooms in religious rites. In modern Western society, they are entertained for their psychedelic effects.

The American banker and amateur mycologist R. Gordon Wasson and his wife Valentina studied the ancient religious practices of the aborigines of a remote settlement in Mexico among which, some of them ingested mushrooms. In 1957 they published an article in the Life magazine entitled "Seeking the Magic Mushroom", in which they described the hallucinatory experiences during those rituals.

Then they were accompanied on another expedition by the French mycologist Roger Heim, director of the National Museum of Natural History of France during this expedition, and it was possible to identify several fungi as Psilocybe species. In turn, Heim also managed to grow the fungus in France and sent some samples to be analysed by the chemist Albert Hofmann, who was working for the

Swiss multinational pharmaceutical company Sandoz.

Hofmann, who had synthesized LSD in 1938, was the first to realize the significance and chemical composition of the purified mixtures he named psilocybin and psilocin. Starting an investigation group that was able to identify and isolate the compounds from Psilocybe Mexicana, Hofmann was helped by his predisposition to ingest mushroom extracts. He and his colleagues then synthesized a certain number of compounds that were chemically similar to natural psilocybin.

The phosphoryl or hydroxy collection to the top of the indole band was transferred to other positions in the band.

Different amounts of methyl groups (CH_3) were added, and other chains carbonized to the side chains and nitrogen in the indole ring to see how these changes could affect psych activity.

Hofmann synthesized two diethyl analogues (two ethyl groups instead of the two methyl groups) of psilocybin and psilocin, 4-phosphoryloxy-N, N-diethyltryptamine, called CY-19 and 4-hydroxy-N, N-diethyltryptamine, called CZ-74. Because their effects lasted approximately three and a half hours (compared to almost twice the time caused by psilocybin), they proved to be more beneficial in European clinics that practised the psychotherapeutic method of "psychotic therapy". Together with controlled drug use, psychedelic Sandoz sold pure psilocybin under the name of *Indocibine* to doctors around the world.

During the early 1960s, Harvard University grew a course of study for psilocybin, into the works of Timothy Leary as well as his colleague Richard Alpert (now known as Ram Dass). Leary was able to obtain synthetic psilocybin from Hofmann through the pharmaceutical company Sandoz (now Novartis). Although a considerable amount of experiments in the early 60s demonstrated positive results of the use of psilocybin in clinical psychiatry, the hysteria of LSD in those times dragged psilocybin with it into the category of Schedule I of illicit drugs in 1970. The 1970s saw the emergence of psilocybin as the "preferred entheogen".

This was due, in part, to broad dissemination of information about it, which was also included in Carlos Castaneda's first book and in several other authors' books that taught the technique for people to cultivate their psilocybin mushrooms on their own. One of the most popular of those books was edited under the pseudonyms of OT Oss and ON Oeric by J. Bigwood, DJ McKenna, K. Harrison

McKenna, and TK McKenna, entitled "*Psilocybin: The Magic Mushroom Grower's Guide*". It sold nearly 100,000 copies by 1981.

These authors adopted the San Antonio technique (for the production of edible fungi by incubating mycelial cultures in a rye substrate; San Antonio 1971) to the output of *Psilocybe [Stropharia] Cubensis*. The new technique requires the use of shared kitchen implements. For the first time, people who were not professionals could produce a potent entheogen in their home, without access to advanced technology, machinery, or chemical equipment.

Spiritual Significance

The knowledge that man has of the hallucinogenic properties of these mushrooms goes back to our ancestors. No one understands for sure when they started to consume hallucinogenic mushrooms, but the most recent period known is that of the Inca and Maya tribes. However, their consumption could be as old as humanity.

These tribes used hallucinogenic mushrooms for healing and spiritual and religious ceremonies. We do not know what injuries, diseases or infections they would have been used for. Some scientists even believe they used hallucinogenic mushrooms to cure mental illness. Only a few years ago, our modern medicine rescued these psychedelic mushrooms again. Some studies prove a very positive influence on people with depressive disorders.

In spiritual ceremonies, hallucinogenic mushrooms were used to make contact with their gods or beyond, and as a way of hearing the voices of their gods during religious rituals. The development of the Inca culture still dates back to the Stone Age, but they had already gained enormous knowledge about the stars, agriculture, martial arts.

Traditional consumption of hallucinogenic mushrooms has been found mainly in America and a few regions of Asia. In Europe, use began in the twentieth century through the hippy generation.

Terence McKenna was a well-known scientist in the hippy era. He studied the ontological foundations of shamanism and the ethnopharmacology of spiritual transformation for three decades. After graduating in Ecology, Resource Conservation and Shamanism from the University of Berkeley, California, he travelled extensively through the tropical regions of Asia and America, thoroughly investigating the shamanic phenomena and ethnomedicine of the Amazon basin. Terence McKenna published more than a dozen books. The strain Psylocibe Cubensis McKenna takes its name from him.

The last and most significant cultural consumption of psychedelic mushrooms was in Indian tribes who lived in America before the Europeans took control. In most cases they were also consumed in religious ceremonies, and a large part of these natives consumed them to talk to people in the hereafter, such as their grandparents, or to obtain support from their spirits and gods.

When modern civilization began its investigation into mescaline in the twentieth century, the spread of other psychedelics such as the hallucinogenic mushrooms grew at the same time. People began to want more psychedelics because each one has unique characteristics in terms of its psychedelic effects. Since those days, the use of hallucinogenic mushrooms has not disappeared again.

For millennium of years, humans have had an intense relationship with psychoactive mushrooms. One way or another, our ancestors found fungi in nature and consumed them.

Psilocybin in the Past

Images have been found in prehistoric murals all over the world that point to the use of hallucinogenic mushrooms thousands of years ago. Antediluvian paintings in caves of the Tassili Plateau, north of Algeria, show amazing images of human figures with fungi that leave their bodies. They have been dated around 5,000 years BC. Later, over 1,000 years BC, we can find cultures native to South America that built temples for the mushroom gods. They also left stone engravings with mushroom shapes, which are believed to have been used in religious ceremonies. Mixtec and Aztec cultures used a series of sacred medicinal plants, such as peyote, sage Divinorum and, of course, fungi, which they called Teonanacatl, the flesh of the gods.

When the Spaniards began the conquest of Central America, in the 16th century, the use of psilocybin was documented for the first time. Alcohol was previously popularly applied, often symbolically in religious acts. Stories of explorers began to arrive praising the use of cacti and hallucinogenic mushrooms in tribal cults. The conquerors described the traditional ceremonies of a spiritual and prophetic nature.

This was unknown in Europe, so conservative attitudes appeared in the Catholic Church, and the mushrooms were declared profane, marginalizing their consumption underground. In 1521, the Aztecs had already been practically dominated, and their population had significantly declined. Catholicism was introduced into their culture, and wisdom about mushrooms almost wholly fell into oblivion.

The First Rebirth

However, some rituals survived the Inquisition, and in 1938, Richard Evans Schultes, known as the father of "ethnobotany", witnessed a traditional sacred mushroom ceremony in Oaxaca, Mexico. The following year he published a report on his experiences at the Botanical Museum of Harvard University.

The first documented explorers who tested the mushrooms were R. Gordon Wasson, a mycologist, and his photographer, Allan Richardson. Wasson learned about the adventures of Schultes and travelled to Mexico in 1955 to see a shaman, Maria Sabina. There, he rediscovered and was invited to a secret fungal ritual. Wasson wrote several books and endorsed that these surviving ceremonies were the evolutions of the same ancestral rites with mushrooms that have inspired many spiritual traditions throughout the world.

During spiritual iconography, we can recognise secret evidence to the use of fungi, encrypted with numerous layers of ancestral gnosis between their images and metaphors. In the East, Vedimos describes a visionary divine sacrament known as Soma. In the West, in Ancient Greece, those attending the Eleusinian Mysteries drank a sacred ritual they called Kykeon. Could it be that all the major religions of this world were inspired by spiritual perceptions obtained through visionary plants?

Wasson's discoveries were published in "Life" magazine in 1957. He had worked hand in hand with Sabina and wrote an article strongly praising the virtues of mushrooms. The term "magic mushroom" was coined, and spread throughout the psychedelic community, motivating Albert Hoffman (the creator of the LSD) to isolate the psilocybin element for distribution in 1956.

Following the Wasson report, Timothy Leary also travelled to Mexico to begin to investigate the phenomenon of fungi. In 1960, he conducted experiments on himself, on Harvard students or on prisoners who volunteered for the cause. Using LSD and magic mushrooms, they claimed to have achieved a recidivism prevention rate of 90%, creating a stir among the media.

The Modern Mushrooms

At present, with the birth of the Internet, information about mushrooms has been extended. Science has shown that psilocin is safe to ingest and that it can have a large number of health benefits. The increase in "smart shops" combined with modern mycological techniques has led to a resurgence of magic mushrooms (a recent study in Denmark stated that about 7% of students had tried them).

Synthetic substitutes for psilocybin have been created in the laboratory, and new organic entheogenic technologies have been developed for modern healers. Could it be that the mushrooms that have always accompanied the human being are the enzyme for the metamorphosis of our mindfulness? Is it likely that this ideal situation that psilocybin gives is the inspiration for a modern global religion?

Biology of psilocybin: Psilobicin is a natural compound that is found in varying concentrations in about 200 species of basidiomycete fungi, mainly among the following genera: *Psilocybe* (116 species), *Gymnopilus* (14 species), *Panaeolus* (13 species), *Copelandia* (12 species), *Hypholoma* (6 species), *Pluteus* (6 species), *Inocybe* (1 species), *Conocybe* (4 species), *Panaeolina* (4 species), *Gerronema* (2 species) and *Agrocybe* (6 species), *Galerina* and *Mycena* (1 species each).

The spores of these fungi do not contain psilocybin or psilocin. The hat of the mushroom tends to have a more significant number of psychoactive compounds than its stem. Total potency varies significantly between species and even between individuals of the same species on the same substrate.

Younger and smaller fungi have a higher concentration of alkaloids and have a milder taste than those more massive and more mature. In general, the psilocybin content in mushrooms is very variable (from almost nothing to about 1.5% of the dry weight of the fungus). It depends on the species, growth and drying conditions, as well as the size of the fungus.

The mature mycelium contains some psilocybin, while the young mycelium (recently germinated from the spores) does not contain considerable amounts of alkaloids. Many species of fungi that contain psilocybin also have small amounts of psilocybin analogues: *Balochistan* and *Norbaeocistin*.

Most species of fungi that contain psilocybin acquire tiny greenish-blue spots (scratches) when handled or damaged due to oxidation of phenolic compounds, oxidation of psilocybin. This result, nonetheless, is not definitive a method used for the identification or determination of the potency of a fungus.

Psilocybin is a prodrug that is pharmacologically converted into the active compound psilocin within the group by a dephosphorylation response. This biochemical effect becomes room below completely acidic circumstances, or also, under the physiological conditions of the body where an enzyme called phosphatase is involved. The oxidation of psilocin by the enzyme hydroxy-indole oxidase gives the dark blue compound ortho - quinone. The latter quickly experiences an electronic transfer, a characteristic that is thought to play an essential role in its physiological activity.

Psilocybin is a tryptamine that has a chemical structure derived from tryptophan that has an indole-like configuration linked to an ethylamine substituent. It has a close structural similarity with the neurotransmitter serotonin (5-

hydroxytryptamine). Psilocybin acts a zwitterionic alkaloid that remains dissoluble in water, moderately dissolvable in methanol as well as ethanol, and insoluble in most natural solvents. Vulnerability to light is detrimental to the stability of the aqueous solutions of psilocybin oxidizing rapidly (a consideration that must be taken into account when used as a standard analytical solution.

A Japanese group described a method for large-scale production of psilocybin without the need for chromatographic purification in the year 2003. The technique, starting with 4-hydroxy-indole psilocybin generated from psilocin, a yield of 85%, a marked increase in returns of synthesis previously published. The psilocybin when purified is a white powder in the form of needles with a melting point between 190°C - 198°C.

Spiritual Effects

The "spiritual" effects of certain hallucinogens persist long after they have been administered. Perhaps, thanks to this type of research, intense religious experiences could be explained, or new treatments developed.

Johns Hopkins scientists show that psilocybin, a substance contained in hallucinogenic mushrooms, produces effects that are interpreted as "spiritual" by those who take it and its psychological impact, which can be construed as beneficial, seem to last more than a year.

In a previous study, carried out by the same team and published in 2006, 36 volunteers participated in a test in which psilocybin was administered under controlled conditions. Now, in the article recently published in the *Journal of Psychopharmacology*, it is said that these people perceived the effects of this substance as positive even 14 months after being exposed to it.

Among the results, they reported feeling good and being more satisfied with their lives. According to Roland Griffiths, one of the researchers participating in the study, most of the volunteers, when evoking the event 14 months ago, describe the experience as the most or one of the universal critical spiritual practices of their lives.

In the article, the researchers give recommendations for this type of study, given the risks that underlie the administration of this type of drug. The fundamental thing is to avoid administering hallucinogens to people at risk of suffering from psychosis or other types of mental disorders. In this way, the researchers provide a guide to prepare patients and provide psychological help during and after the psychedelic experience (lasting 8 hours).

These practices would contribute both to "travel" safety and to the standardization of the protocol in this type of research. Mathew W. Johnson says that, with proper filtering and patient preparation, hallucinogens can have a level of safety comparable to other medicines used in research or medical procedures.

Remember that decades ago LSD (another hallucinogen) was used in medical research, which is what it had been designed for, but since the sixties, the reputation of these types of drugs plummeted due to the excesses of the time. The profusion of its use as a recreational drug broke this type of investigation once the substance was banned.

Psilocybin is an alkaloid that exerts its action on some brain receptors that generally respond to the neurotransmitter serotonin. Certain cultures have used certain fungi that contain this alkaloid for hundreds of years for religious reasons.

In the 2006 study (published in Psychopharmacology) 36 volunteers participated with a proper cultural level and leading active spiritual lives. 60% of them said that their contact with psilocybin was a mystical experience. The experience consisted of, as they relate, in the sense of the existence of a higher truth or a feeling of unity.

After fourteen months, the researchers passed a questionnaire to these same volunteers. The results show that the same proportion of volunteers rated their experience as the most or one of the most significant of their lives and said it also had increased their sense of well-being or satisfaction with life.

According to Griffiths, hallucinogens could provide a method to investigate the neurological basis of religious experiences by invoking in the laboratory the same type of mystical experiences that can be had through meditation, prayer or the like. These researchers also want to test the effect of these types of drugs on atheists or agnostics.

According to Griffiths, the finding is significant, since psychological research rarely reports such persistent results from a single laboratory event. This would give credibility to those who suggest that the mystical experiences, which some people have during a session with hallucinogens, can help patients suffering from anxiety or depression due to diseases such as cancer, and serve as potential treatments for others' dependencies.

Usually, these types of patients receive healthy doses of analgesics, antidepressants and anxiolytics.

If you could change your perception of death and reduce your stress with hallucinogens instead of the usual system, you could improve your quality of life. These researchers will study this possible application.

Griffiths notes that while one party reported having passed fear or anxiety at some time during the session, none said they had suffered prolonged harmful effects. Nor was there any clinical evidence that indicated the existence of injury of any kind.

Researchers warn, however, that if hallucinogens are misused, possible fear or anxiety responses can lead to harmful behaviours.

A single take of psilocybin can help calm down efficiently, and for several months, two diseases that are, at the same time, two epidemics of the modern world. At least that is what two research published recently in the *"Journal of Psychopharmacology"* say.

The problem is that this active principle is part of the hallucinogenic mushrooms, so the controversy is served. Fungi that possess psilocybin are generally used as a drug for recreational purposes or spiritual purposes, within the practices of some religions and sects. Let us avoid, in any case, facing the issue from prejudice and see, then, what such investigations say.

The Medicine of Happiness

The surprising conclusions appear after psilocybin has been administered to patients affected by a disease as distressing and aggressive as cancer.

About 40% of people diagnosed with some type of tumour suffer from anxiety or depression. Antidepressants in these cases have limited effects, particularly as regards the existential aspect. Many of those affected come to conceive of life as meaningless, opening up for them, in certain circumstances, to the terrible possibility of suicide.

Psilocybin produced a surprising increase in the quality of life and mood of the patients.

In work carried out by scientists from the University of New York, 19 patients who were in an advanced state of the disease were divided into two groups. Both followed a supportive psychological therapy, but one of them took a single dose of 0.3 milligrams of psilocybin for every kilo of body weight. The other group, on the other hand, followed a treatment based on vitamin B3.

After seven weeks, the substances were exchanged between the participants.

According to the authors, the results were: "fast, reliable and well-founded". Single doses dramatically reduced depression and anxiety levels for more than seven weeks, maintaining its effects for up to eight months after taking it.

The second study is based on the work of a group of doctors from the John Hopkins University of Medicine. Fifty-one patients with advanced cancer were also divided into two sets: at first, each was given either a therapeutic dose or a low dose of psilocybin. Five weeks later, the proportions were exchanged.

When the experience was over, fear and anxiety were gone, and my life had changed.

As in the research carried out by the University of New York, psilocybin produced a significant increase in their quality of life, a higher capacity to accept death and an increase in optimism in the sick.

"As an atheist, it is complicated for me to say this, but it was as if I were bathed in the love of God", says Dinah Bazer, one of the patients undergoing treatment, in statements to 'Bloomberg'. "This feeling lasted hours. When the experience was over, the fear and anxiety were gone, and my life had changed".

Several of the patients said that taking psilocybin ended up restructuring their minds. Some even used the word "mystic" to describe their feelings. Still, scientists involved in the experiments, such as Professor Roland Griffiths from John Hopkins University, say they want to run away from these controversies. Griffiths confesses to the newspaper *The Guardian*: "Sounds like a little scientist. It seems that we were postulating other mechanisms beyond neuroscience, and I am not defending this".

Other researchers involved, such as Dr Stephen Ross, director of the addiction department of the University of New York, show less reluctance when talking about the experiences described by the individuals studied.

"We have a small system that, when you tickle it, produces these states of alteration that have been described as spiritual or mystical states in different religions. They have also been defined as unity states. People feel that the separation that exists between their ego and the outside world dissolves and they think that they are part of energy or a state of continuous consciousness linked to the universe".

A Taboo to Overcome?

Hallucinogenic mushrooms are usually included among the list of very dangerous narcotics. These lists, according to David Nutt, a specialist in neuropsychopharmacology at Imperial College London, are an official convention, because there is no direct relationship between the actual classification of drugs and the damage they cause.

According to Nutt, the reality is that many narcotics treated as taboo are not as harmful to the consumer as compared to other drugs that pose significant health risks such as heroin, crack, methamphetamine, cocaine or alcohol.

The two studies on psilocybin come to light a few days after the "US Food and Drug Administration" approved a series of experiments with ecstasy, to study their therapeutic possibilities in patients affected by post-traumatic stress disorder.

Already in the 60s, LSD, ecstasy or psilocybin offered, for many psychiatrists, new and exciting medical perspectives. The strict anti-narcotic laws that emerged, however, during the 1970s were an obstacle to investigations. Scientists interested in their possibilities have since had to fight against legal, ethical and cultural difficulties to reopen options for experimenting with them.

Psilocybin Is Extracted from Hallucinogenic Mushrooms

"I think it's a big issue, both for the results and in historical terms. All this was, at the time, part of psychiatry and is now returning to today" - Dr Ross points out.

Unfortunately, the adverse aspects of drugs have been affected too much, and the benefits that can be extracted from them have been forgotten.

Nutt points out: "One of my challenges, in the rest of my career, is that these drugs be re-investigated because, for example, I am sure that ecstasy is very useful for people with disorders caused by chronic stress. Psilocybin is also useful against migraines and resistant depression. Finally, LSD serves to treat dying patients, and helps them cope with the experience of death".

The dilemma about the use of these narcotics can change if the moral conflict arises from another perspective. In an annexe that accompanies the studies, Craig Blinderman, director of the palliative care unit of the Presbyterian Hospital in New York, warns that several countries are legislating to allow people to end their pain through euthanasia. What would happen if psilocybin could not only relieve the existential anguish of these patients, but also provide purpose to the days of those in a final state?

Nutt points out how inhuman the therapies that are being used in some palliative care units can be: "What we do today is poison them with opioids, so their mind is already dead. They die without really knowing what is happening".

Psilocybin, a compound that contains magic mushrooms, has healing properties already exploited by ancestral cultures. Now scientists, despite legal obstacles, try it to treat diseases such as depression or anxiety.

The compound that contains magic mushrooms and that causes the hallucinogenic effects, and psilocybin has powerful properties that ancient cultures have already exploited as a medicinal remedy, and that now scientists have begun to try to treat depression, migraines, anxiety because of cancer and addiction to drugs such as alcohol or cocaine.

However, investigating with magic mushrooms, even in a clinical setting, today has significant legal obstacles, and the few researchers who dare to examine with it must go through a long and expensive pilgrimage.

A few months ago, in the United Kingdom, at Imperial College, London, a clinical trial to give psilocin to 12 patients with depression was just started. "Although from the outset they had the money to carry out the investigation, they had to wait three years to obtain the relevant authorizations and that the extract from the only authorized laboratory in the world authorized to distribute it legally arrived", he explained to VICE News David Nutt, head of the neuropsychopharmacology unit at Imperial College.

"Psilocybin, if administered in a controlled manner, in a clinical setting and with the appropriate doses, can "reconfigure" the brains of people with depression and eliminate the loop of negative thoughts that feedback the disease", explains Nutt.

In an earlier study, Nutt and Robin Carhart-Harris, a researcher at the same center, used magnetic resonance imaging to enter the brain during the psychedelic journey and see what changed. They observed that psilocin suppresses activity in one area, the medial prefrontal cortex, usually hyperactive in people suffering from depression.

"It also acts in the production of serotonin, a neurotransmitter that people with depression produce in smaller quantities" Magí Farré, head of the Clinical Pharmacology Service of the Germans Trias I Pujol Hospital, located in the Spanish city of Badalona, tells VICE News.

"In low doses, it is believed that it may have therapeutic potential", he says. On the other hand, this natural hallucinogen has an evocative power that "would also allow recovering memories to work in them", adds Farré.

God in a Pill

In the United States, a research group at John Hopkins University has been testing its effectiveness in smoking cessation and so that terminal cancer patients face the inevitable journey to death in the best way. The participants in this latest study were able to change the experience thanks to the mystical experience that doctors induced with the intake of psilocybin. They managed to reduce the anguish and thus provide a sweeter ending. Some have even come to baptize psilocybin as "God in a pill".

Along the same lines, another group from the University of New York is about to start the third phase of trials with a large number of terminal cancer patients. As if they were masters of ceremonies, doctors guide the patient during the taking and the duration of its effect. Upon awakening, his perception has changed; his anguish has transformed. Very few are those who suffer the worst of the side effects that can have: the agony of a bad trip.

Traditional Medicine

The therapeutic use of psilocybin is nothing new. In different cultures, traditional medicine has used them to heal. From the Aztec civilization, through the popular María Sabina in Mexico, even healers of the same Iberian Peninsula just 20 years ago, according to a study by Juan Andrés Oria de Rueda, professor of mycology at the University of Valladolid, in which he has collected testimonies of older women who in the past trained as healers in Extremadura, Ávila and Zamora.

"These types of fungi have been used primarily for headaches, these are widespread native species in Spain, such as the *Psilocybe semilanceata*, to those who called Fungueiru or Mushroom of Aunt Juana, and who are very present in grassland areas, because they grow mainly thanks to the droppings of cattle", Oria de Rueda explains to VICE News. "His interest is to try them for treating cluster migraines, which are headaches so intense that there have even been cases in which they have led to suicide", explains Oria.

Amanita muscaria, which contains other hallucinogenic substances, such as *muscimol* and *ibotenic acid* "are the best known, but have different effects", Oria points out.

Against the Ban

Psychedelic substances, both LSD and psilocybin, were used in clinical psychiatry research until after 1971, after United Nations Convention on Psychotropic Substances, they were gradually banned worldwide, James Rucker, a specialist tells VICE News.

Psilocybin can reconfigure the brains of people with depression and eliminate the loop of negative thoughts.

This British psychiatrist defends the need to give more facilities permission to research with these substances, to the point that he has made a banner by publishing the prestigious British Medical Journal, with an article in which he asks for the requalification of these substances for scientific use.

He's not the only one. David Nutt, who has suffered a long bureaucratic path to get to do his clinical trials to treat depression, has also published another report article in PLOS Biology this year. He has found it very difficult to obtain the necessary permits by the European Union and the British government. He also denounces the control of the sale of psilocybin by the only laboratory that produces it.

In addition to the legal obstacles and the difficulty for the ethical committees to approve it, in the case of psilocybin there is an economic brake, Rucker explains. "Because of the restrictions established by the United Nations, there is only one manufacturer in the world that produces psilocybin of sufficient quality to be used in these studies, at a prohibitive price of more than 130,000 Euros per gram, which gives 50 doses", says Rucker.

In the United Kingdom, also, the government requires authorized research groups to pay a license for this activity amounting to more than 6,000 Euros. Besides, the permit takes at least one year to arrive.

False Myths

According to the psychiatrist at King's College, the authorities of the moment built false myths around psychotropics, such as inciting suicide.

According to a meta-analysis of the scientific studies carried out before the prohibition of these substances and using controlled doses, there is no risk of suicide or self-harm. Unlike other drugs, it is not addictive.

Some see in the ban an apparent attempt to dismantle the counterculture of the time. It was chemist Albert Hoffman who managed to synthesize for the first time in a laboratory a hallucinogen, LSD, in 1947, and 11 years later, psilocybin, in 58. But it was an article published a year earlier in Life magazine by one who made the magic mushrooms famous, in which Robert Wasson, a banker and ethnologist who independently researched, that explained the psychedelic experiences he lived through on a trip to the mountains.

From there, psilocin left the clinical setting, and different movements began to experiment with psychedelic drugs, among them mushrooms. The same day that Kennedy took the presidency of the United States, Jack Kerouac himself tested laboratory psilocybin (which was then produced by Sandoz), as narrated in a letter addressed to Timothy Leary, a psychologist who at that time devoted himself to extensive research. With these substances. The hippy movement also endorsed the psychedelic arsenal.

In addition to psilocybin, scientists are interested in being able to investigate other hallucinogens. LSD also seems to be effective in anxiety and migraines, and ecstasy could be used to treat post-traumatic stress.

Spiritual Use of Giant Mushroom

Far from the recreational connotation is the spiritual. Although they are linked to the culture of a people, the meaning and depth of the consumption of sacred plants in indigenous societies are much more profound.

Shamans are considered wise and visionary. They use various techniques that vary depending on the tribe. Sometimes the mind captures the images that come through dreams or visions, while in others, these visualizations are instead induced, which are known as rituals.

The shamans rituals have as their fundamental characteristic the intake of psychotropic substances (fungi and plants) that they consider as sacred plants. But it is not merely that, but it is accompanied by other techniques of meditation, stimulation of perception, dances, and music. With all this, they reach a state of consciousness that allows them to guide their people, visualize the future, establish contact with God that will help them on the way forward, and acquire healing properties.

All this is produced by the conception of the world that the indigenous people have that life is formed by different planes of reality, that they are interconnected and that only shamans are capable, due to the gifts they have been granted, to see and understand.

This way of understanding the world is what is called worldview, consisting of five planes of reality: totality, energy, communion, sacredness, and community sense of life. Five spheres that can only be understood by the shamans in their rituals, in which the sacred plants are essential to be able to travel through the different worlds and thus establish the bonds of the union that helps them to understand.

A group of figurines in central Guatemala were interpreted as mushroom stems dating back to 500 BC. One ancestral tradition in which the shamans of many indigenous tribes of South America continue to use these hallucinogenic mushrooms. They are considered as 'sacred plants' to heal the soul, cure diseases, or know the future in the book of life. Carlos Martínez, an Argentine anthropologist prominent in original research, states that the

Foundation's team from America that he directs calls that these robust medicinal plants are sacred whose origin dates back thousands of years. Discarding the term "hallucinogens" because it has pathological connotations that do not correspond to the use and effects of those plants.

Therefore, it is possible to establish whether hallucinogenic fungi and therefore plants, are or are not a drug. As Juan José Llopis, a professor at the Jaume I University of Castellón in the department of psychobiology, explains, the concept of drugs is given instead of the purpose for which the substance is used. The correct connotation is that of 'sacred mushrooms', and in that context, in the ritual of the ancestral ceremonies of the Amazonian tribes, it does not have the drug connotation. Instead, when the context is recreational use, that is when they become a drug.

It is known that there are currently in America, Europe, and Asia, about seventy fungi that contain psilocin and psilocybin, two substances that modify cognitive processes, moods, or even perceptions. The European countries where hallucinogenic mushrooms are most consumed are Spain (Basque Country, Navarra, Catalonia, and the Valencian Community), the Netherlands, and England.

And the most common acquisition mode is through the Internet. Ana Maria Lopez, psychologist and sexologist in the city of Linares that collaborates with the Association of Rehabilitated Alcoholics of the municipality believes that easy access to the sale of substances online is very harmful and should restrict its use and control access to people over 18 as in the case of medications.

In the case of Holland, it is not until recently, in 2007, when the explicit prohibition of the consumption of hallucinogenic mushrooms is established. Its use was so every day that many coffee shops made pies with mushrooms and served it to the citizens in addition to the sale in the so-called 'Smart shops', of the new variant. However, the government decided after a successive wave of incidents and even the death of a young man, to end the tolerance and to avoid the arrival of tourists, who are already looking for cannabis.

In the accessible version, mushrooms in our country can be purchased as well on the Internet, but also by word of mouth, as many of the drugs are sold in cities. Those who have consumed it recommend to each other that it is better to do it in a group in an enclosed place, but under the watchful eye of someone who has not taken them, since some of the trances can cause someone to jump into an open window, believing, for example, that they were thrown into a pool.

There is a reoccurring of interest in the use of psychedelic drugs as a form of management for emotional suffering secondary to terminal cancer. In particular, the effect of a compound found in the so-called "magic mushrooms", that is, psilocybin has been studied. Single doses of psilocybin would appear to induce beneficial effects on the way of feeling and perceiving, fostering the ability to generate new associations and meanings in such a way that, in theory, there would be a re-consolidation of the existential purpose taken away by the fear of death.

Without pretending to be an expert in the subject of thanatology, I think that specific changes in psychological dynamics will occur in the face of death. For example, it has been speculated that "positive illusions" are an integral part of homeostasis of mental well-being, and there is little doubt that two of the components of positive illusions would be hampered in patients with terminal cancer: optimistic bias and illusion of control, respectively, the preference of believing that we have a lower risk of experiencing negative experiences than others, and the tendency to overestimate one's ability to control events.

Without the possibility of keeping minimum positive expectations regarding the immediate future, and with significant problems to project ourselves in time (except to anticipate a painful agony), we would easily fall into what some consider a state of "spiritual distress", or even "spiritual deficit". That is an acute lack of purpose, meaning, and the possibilities of self-transcendence.

"Spiritual" is, of course, a non-scientific terminology, and therefore in my inappropriate opinion, its use outside the religious sphere. Attempts to investigate the use of psilocybin as a way to alleviate the terror of death is an excellent way to highlight the problems that arise when considering this "spiritual dimension" in the equation.

Already in 1962 Walter Pahnke and Timothy Leary were studying spiritual, mystical and religious experiences in volunteers who were administered psychedelics. They reported that the psilocybin group said they had significantly more profound religious experiences than the control group. This could suggest that the therapeutic is secondary to the increase of religiosity, or a renewed faith in the supernatural.

I believe that regardless of personal ideology, for scientific research purposes, terms with this type of connotations are not necessary, although it must be admitted that in the investigation of the therapeutic use of psychedelics. It is not very easy to completely stop using the concept of the spiritual. The neurochemically active compound derived from it (psilocin) stabilizes the mood and seems to facilitate the rehabilitation of the "sense of purpose" and self-transcendence. Psilocin is a chemically similar compound - almost identical - to serotonin, stimulating with particular potency a variety of serotonin receptors: 5HT2 RL Carhart-Harris et al.

They speculate from a neuro-psychoanalytic approach that psilocybin acts by dissolving the functions of the ego - the self-referential services - that it considers dependence on the so-called Default Network). The Natural Network is a set of brain areas that are particularly active when we let our minds wander typically valued in research with Functional Magnetic Resonance by closing the eyes or fixing the gaze on a cross.

Leaving most of the brain regions that conform it located in the medial part of our brain: Posterior Cortex of the Cingulum, Anterior Cortex of the Cingulum, Cortex Fronto-Medial, Medial Temporal Lobes. Additionally, areas of the Temporo-Parietal Junction that have been associated with the ability to infer the intentions of others (Theory of Mind) are added. Carhart-Harris identifies this neuro-circuit with Freudian Secondary Processes.

Interestingly, in Cotard Syndrome, patients who deliriously claim to be dead, there is, in fact, an extreme hip functionality of the Default Network (see "Interview with a Dead Man" in NewScientist). It can then be theorized that this surprising statement is not, after all, so far-fetched and that what the patient is perceiving is the "death of the ego", and possibly a relative lack of content of consciousness.

Carhart-Harris studied in a later publication (Neural Correlates of the Psychedelic State Determined by the FMRI Under the Effect of Psilocybin) the changes in cortical activity during the intake of psilocybin, and according to the author what was striking was the decrease in cortical activity of regions that act as a procedural crossroads (hubs), and that interconnect distant neural centers.

It is known that the thalamus acts as a filter, so it would be anticipated that a decrease in its function could abnormally increase the number of stimuli that reach the cerebral cortex. Possibly the dissolution of the ego, and therefore of the secondary processes referred to by Freud, is also due to acute failure of these areas (hubs) where processes of different neural levels converge, particularly an induced dysfunction of the Posterior Kindle Cortex. In summary, we have a panorama where the neural correlates of the ego are dysfunctional due to this potent agonist of the 5HT2 serotonin receptors, and where the incoming sensory information hyper stimulates the cerebral cortex.

One more reflection. If this speculative line is correct, during the state induced by psilocybin, the processes that are substrates of Magic Thought could be released, and that correspond to the primary methods described by Freud.

The perception of agency, not already restricted by the mechanisms of the ego or by the Default Network, would seem to invade sense-perception. That is, psilocybin would induce an abnormal state of hyper-mentalism that largely explains the phenomenology observed, in addition to understanding why this drug has been classified within the group of entheogens. Hyper mentalism acts as a conductive thread that makes it easy to find the lost purpose in patients with terminal illnesses, taking proper care of the environmental variables during therapeutic consumption, in addition to a subsequent psychotherapeutic follow-up. In successful cases, the drug seems to facilitate a kind of "reconnection" with others, with external reality, with our past, and with our feelings.

Recovering the meaning and purpose for one's existence is the desired result of these interventions and, as I said, is catalyzed by induced hypermetabolism. The liberation of Magic Thought enables the healing of the "spiritual deficit" referred to frequently. On the other hand, with the sharp decrease in the activity of the Medial Pre-Frontal Brain, the hyperactivity of cortical areas that have been associated with depressive disorder disappears. Somehow, and despite the proximity of death, the illusions, biases, and emotions so necessary for psychological well-being can be partially recovered. A valid "reset" of the ability to be happy.

Psilocybin can induce mystical experiences of personal and spiritual significance. For example, in the Marsh Chapel Experiment, led by graduate student Walter Pahnke at Harvard Divinity School under the supervision of Timothy Leary. Almost all of the seminary graduates who received psilocybin reported having had deeply spiritual experiences. After 25 years of the experiment, all those subjects to whom psilocybin was administered in it described their experience as "of a genuine mystical nature and characterized it as one of the highest moments of their spiritual life".

Rick Doblin considered the original study partially defective due to an incorrect implementation of the double-blind method. In addition to several wrong questions in the questionnaire. He argues that this study suggests "considerable doubt about the claim that mystical experiences catalyzed by drugs are by no means inferior to mystical experiences without drugs both in their immediate content and in their long-term effects".

In 2006, a group of researchers from the Johns Hopkins School of Medicine conducted by Roland R. Griffiths experimented to determine the degree of mystical experience and the effects of attitude in the course of experience induced by the psilocybin. This, through the use of a modified version of the questionnaire and with a more rigorous double-blind.

Various experts supported the study for the strength of their experimental design in the evaluation of the psychological effects produced by the ingestion of psilocybin. In the experiment, psilocybin and methylphenidate were administered (Ritalin) in separate sessions to 36 volunteers without previous experience with hallucinogens, and the methylphenidate sessions served as a control and the same as a placebo substance.

The degree of mystical experience was measured by using a questionnaire about the mystical experiences developed by Ralph W. Hood; 61% of the subjects reported a "complete mystical experience" after the psilocybin session, while only 13% reported the same result in the methylphenidate sessions. Two months after the intake of psilocybin, 79% of the participants said they had moderately or significantly increased their sense of well-being.

Around 36% of the participants also had a "scary experience" dysphoria (that is, a bad trip during the psilocybin session that was not reported by any subject during the methylphenidate session), with about a third of them (13% of the total) who claimed that the dysphoria dominated the entire course.

Such adverse effects were easily managed by the researchers and did not have a lasting negative impact on the feeling of well-being of the subjects. Subsequent measurements at 14 months of the experience confirmed that the participants continued to assign deep personal meaning to the experience.

Later studies of this same group investigated the relationship between the dose of psilocybin with the probability of a mystical experience in healthy volunteers. A double-blind study showed that psychedelic mushrooms could give people an encounter with significant personal and spiritual significance. In such a study, one-third of the subjects reported that ingestion of psychedelic mushrooms was the most spiritually significant time of their lives, and about two-thirds said it among the five most critical spiritual functions of their lives.

On the other hand, one-third of the subjects said they had extreme anxiety. Related research conducted by this same group looks for whether the mystical experiences in volunteers who are given psilocybin can help with anxiety and mood caused by cancer. In 2017 a study showed that psilocybin experiences brought more lasting positive changes when combined with regular meditation.

There was only one reported case that psilocybin and cannabis probably caused a persistent hallucinogenic perceptual disorder; although recent clinical studies do not show such side effects.

Relationship to Humanity

This substance incorporated into the body, modifies the affectivity, the relationship with the environment, and behaviour. Depending on the dose, intermittent psycho-sensory phenomena can occur. It provides a visionary state of consciousness and an increase in perception.

The primary effects of oral intake of one gram of these fungi last on average four to six hours. Some of the results can range from an absolute hilarity, disinhibition or loquacity, through visual and auditory hallucinations to deeper and new perspectives of reality, time, and space. The physical effects go through an increase in body temperature, gastrointestinal disturbances, especially nausea and vomiting, perceptual disorders and loss of balance.

How to Extract Psilocybin

The exact dose to perceive the entheogenic effects that make him famous depends on several factors, such as the person's metabolism, his fasting state, his mood, his context, and, of course, the concentration of psilocybin in the fungus. A small dose can cause, after about thirty minutes after ingestion, bring a feeling of physical relaxation usually associated with states of transient tranquillity, fatigue, and changes in the perception of the environment. After an hour, most people who ingest the fungus claim to have an inner clarity that allows them to see nature more clearly: auras in flowers and people, trees with more vivid green, and the sky and sunsets as they would never see them in a state of ordinary consciousness.

If the dose is large, the effects are usually much more marked: experiencing hilarity, changes in the notion of time, difficulty in muscle control, and an abnormal interpretation of the information of the senses.

If the dose is intermediate, a combination of these effects may occur.

This type of substance does not carry proven psychological sequelae. Even so, it has been experienced in its therapeutic use against depression, chronic pain, and stress with positive results. In psychopathologies such as schizophrenia, its effects can be dangerous. Experimentation with this and other entheogenic substances is painful to carry out due to a large number of legal restrictions.

Analytical Methods

Many techniques are used to analytical identify and measure the amount of psilocybin in fungi. Some of these techniques are:

- Thin-layer chromatography
- Gas chromatography coupled to mass spectrometry (GC-MS)
- Spectroscopy ion mobility
- Capillary electrophoresis
- Ultraviolet-visible spectroscopy
- Infrared Spectroscopy
- High-performance liquid chromatography (HPLC) with ultraviolet detection methods, by fluorescence, electrochemical, or by using an electrospray in mass spectrometry

The first technique used gas chromatography; however, the problem was that with this method, psilocybin was dephosphorylated to psilocin before carrying out the analysis complicating it.

Several chromatographic techniques have been improved to recognize psilocin in body solutions. *Rapid Emergency Drug Identification*

System (REMEDi HS) is an HPLC-based drug screening method; HPLC with electrochemical detection; GC-MS; and liquid chromatography coupled with mass spectrometry.

Although the determination of urine psilocin levels can be performed without purification of the sample, plasma or serum analysis requires an extraction previous followed by a derivation of the extracts in the case of GC-MS. A specific immunoassay for the detection of psilocin in whole blood samples has also been developed.

A publication during the year 2009 described the separation of forensic importance illicit drugs (psilocybin and psilocin as) using HPLC at high speed became identifiable within 0.5 min of analysis.

Pharmacology

The dephosphorylated psilocybin to psilocin acts as an agonist partial to various receptors of serotonin. Psilocin has a high affinity for the serotonin 5-HT 2A receptor in the brain where it mimics the effects of serotonin. Psilocin binds with less affinity to other serotonergic receptors such as 5-HT 1A 5-HT 1D and 5-HT 2C.

These serotonergic receptors interact with pyramidal neurons in the cerebral cortex, which are believed to be involved in the perception of pain and anxiety. The psychomimetic effects of psilocin can be blocked by the administration of drugs such as ketanserin and risperidone that are antagonists of the 5-HT 2A receptor. Structural analogues of psilocybin and psilocin are used for the structural and functional determination of the coupled receptor.

What Are Magic Mushrooms?

Psilocybin Mushrooms

Psilocybin mushrooms, also called hallucinogenic mushrooms, are fungi that contain psychoactive substances such as *psilocybin*, *psilocin* and *baeocistine*, among others.

There are two types:

Mushrooms with Psilocybin/Psilocin

Mushrooms containing the hallucinogens psilocybin or psilocin are mainly characterized by the following genera: *Psilocybe*, *Stropharia*, *Conocybe* and *Panaeolus*.

Amanita Muscaria

Amanita muscaria does not have psilocybin or psilocin, the hallucinogenic compounds that compose it are *muscimol* and *ibotenic* acid.

The Hallucinogenic Truffles

Apart from their appearance, there is no difference between magic mushrooms and magic truffles. The so-called truffles are not authentic (such as those belonging to the genus Tuber, such as black truffles sold as a delicacy in restaurants and markets), but sclerotia* of psilocybe mushrooms that grow below the ground). Both contain the hallucinogenic molecules of psilocybin, psilocin and baeocistine, and both are entirely effective.

* Definition 1: A sclerotium is a compressed mass of solid mycelium that contains food reserves. The role of sclerotia is to survive in extreme environmental periods.

*Definition 2: Sclerocio - structure of fungal origin, of hard consistency and developed for resistance to unfavourable conditions, germinates in favourable conditions.

It can also appear in myxomycetes.

Where are they?

Habitats

The main types of habitats are:
- Pastures, meadows, or pastures
- Estercoleros
- Banks, gardens and lands removed (rubble)
- Forests

Grasslands or Pastures

This is a typical habitat of humid areas and low altitude. Here appears a large part of the species with a conical hat and thin foot/stem, such as *Psilocybe semilanceata, Ps. Mexican, Ps. strictipes* and others.

Estercoleros

These are species that grow directly on mammalian droppings. Therefore, there is no need to give great explanations. There are species of animals that are more favourable, such as cattle and horses, but even on elephant droppings, Psilocybes appear.

In this type of habitat, there are both psychoactive fungi (*Psilocybe cubensis* and *Panaeoulus cyanescens*), and non-psychoactive-fungi (*Psilocybe coprophilia* or *Ps. Merdaria*) and one of the main characteristics of it is its short life, which takes the stool to decompose.

They grow in gardens, riverbanks, and debris (removed lands), The gardens are an excellent place for the development of psycho-biblical species since they contain decomposing waste and materials. In manure-rich gardens, it is possible to find *Panaeoulus subbalteatus* in temperate zones and *Panaeoulus cyanescens* in tropical areas. Species may also appear as *Psilocybe cyanescens*, *Ps. stuntzii*, *Ps. Baeocystis*, *Ps. caerulescens* and *Ps. subaeruginous* among others.

The riverbanks are open and sunny areas, so it is likely to find some of the species that occur in debris-removed lands. The appearance of fungi in these habitats is due to the floodwaters of the river, and the sediments that are deposited, with numerous wastes of trees or plants, are sandy.

A reasonably potent species that appears in this habitat is *Psilocybe azurescens*, a species discovered by the psilocycological sage, Paul Stamets.

The dumps or rather the removed lands are a habitat where it will be quite natural for us to find some species of Psilocybe. Some examples can be recent works of roads or highways that are built-in forests or similar areas, also an area of recent construction with its consequent earthworks, as well as landslides and natural landslides due to rain or other causes.

Forest

This category is the one that includes the most significant number of species of all those described above. Although due to the considerable variation of parameters, altitude, humidity, and rainfall that exists, each area will have its small catalogue of fungi, among which we will find some Psilocybes.

Perhaps where it is easier to find them is in the forest of certain conifers or deciduous trees (which produce litter and decomposition of it) such as poplar, willow, alder, and others.

Psychoactive mushrooms in Spain: there are eight recognized species of the genus psilocybe in Spain. It is quite probably and even sure there are more species, or some user knows them, but their existence is "officially" unknown.

As hallucinogenic, only three species stand out:

Psilocybe Semilanceata

The queen of the psilocybes is a species quite dominant and highly distributed throughout the globe.

Psilocybe Hispanica

Species endemic to the Pyrenean region (both on the Spanish and French side), were recently discovered by a Spanish researcher (Ignacio Seral-Bozal). It is a coprophile species - that grows directly on the shit or the manure - relatively strange since it grows between 1,500 and 2,300 m of altitude and develops even with very low temperatures or snow.

Psilocybe Gallaeciae

Species of recent discovery. At the moment, it is only known in Galicia (Northwest of Spain) and belongs to the Mexican section, being very similar to this, and it is the first species of this section that was discovered in Europe.

Other psychoactive species

There are several more species of Psilocybe, but they have not been shown to have psychoactive properties, or there is no conclusive data on the content of alkaloids or active ingredients that drive us to think on the possibility of an entheogenic use of that species.

It is also quite probable, by some references, that several Panaeoulus (*Panaeolus subbalteatus*) and Psilocybes can be found on the Iberian Peninsula as *Psilocybe strictipes, Ps. cyanescens*.

How to Get Hallucinogenic Mushrooms

The black market

The black market or so-called submerged market represents 11% of GDP, in addition to accounting for more than 1.8 billion jobs concerning those jobs that are not declared. Also, in our country, there are numerous activities of this nature such as the sale of drugs, prostitution, the manufacture and distribution of counterfeit goods and the piracy of material subject to intellectual property rights that usually develop in our economy and that they represent a high percentage of undeclared income.

The most significant risks are:

- You do not know what they are giving you, and it can be a poisonous mushroom that someone has taken in the field and wants to sell it as a hallucinogen. First of all, find out and guarantee that the seller is trustworthy.

- The product may not be in good condition, either rotten or contaminated, not being suitable for health.
- The dose may not be adequate and may be different for each person. If you buy on the black market, make sure you weigh your dose well with a precision scale.
- That the product is given to you in powder, without being able to distinguish the composition, mushrooms are delivered whole or otherwise broken to reach the dose, but NEVER powdered. If they do so, make sure the powder is mushrooms/truffles, observing the crushing process.

Presentation

They can be sold in the form of a mushroom, fresh or dried, in the way of sclerotia (truffles) or dry powder (sometimes encapsulated).

The amount of psychoactive substances present determines their potency and varies with the species, the variety, the place of growth of the fungus, and the growing conditions.

Obtaining Hallucinogenic

Truffles Hallucinogenic or sclerotia truffles can be obtained in GrowShops, or Smart Shops specialized in the legal form in many countries of Europe. They are presented fresh, and vacuum packed ready to be consumed.

They can also be obtained online, most of the time with the same presentation, and reliably in the best known online stores.

There is no problem with your shipments to private homes and usually come two rations of medium effect for an approximate price of 15 Euros.

Dangers and Advice on the Natural Collection of Hallucinogenic Mushrooms

It is recommended not to go out to the field without previous experience and less the consumption of the found copies. If you want to consume them, get informed, and take them under your responsibility. Still, it is best to go to a mycological association that will advise and certify the name of the specimen found.

In the Peninsula, the most representative and most collected mushrooms for psychonautic use are the Amanita muscaria (the flycatcher mushroom), with a red hat with white speckles, a ring and a white foot, famous for its iconography represented for hundreds of years and its familiarity with Dwarf mushrooms.

The second most collected is the *Psilocybe semilanceata*, of higher potency and high in psilocybin and psilocin. Inquire well before consuming them, although these two mentioned are easy to identify, and rarely can lead to errors, even so, insist that if you are not 100% sure, then it is better not to consume it.

Psilocybe Semilanceata

- **Hat**: 2.5-5 cm. in diameter, from conical to flared.
- **Colour**: From dark brown to yellowish depending on age and humidity. Very viscous if the ambient humidity is high.
- **Blades**: The light colour of young that changes to brown and grey as it matures.
- **Foot**: 40-100 mm long by 0.7-2 mm. Thick and very long and winding: The hats usually appear above the grass. It has no ring.
- **Spore colour**: Dark purple-brown.
- **Habitat and distribution**: It grows in grasslands and grasslands where there is cow or horse manure. It never grows directly on guano. The season is from late summer to fall. In the Iberian Peninsula they only appear in mountain meadows of the mountain ranges of the northern half.
- **Psychoactivity**: The level of active substances can vary between 0.2% and 2.37%, that is, from moderately active to extremely potent.
- **Dosage**: Fresh Dried - Low Dose From 8 to 10 grams, from 0.8 to 1 gram. Average Dose is from

10 to 20 grams, from 1 to 2 grams, High Dose is from 20 to 30 grams, from 2 to 3 grams.

- **Attention**: There are varieties of semilanceata (e.g., Dutch) that are slightly more powerful than those mentioned.

- **Observations**: Known as Money, it is collected in autumn. It contains very little psilocin and a lot of psilocybin, which means that it can be preserved for a long time since psilocybin is very resistant to oxidation. It is a mighty dry species, if we compare it with others of everyday consumption.

Mushroom Products

Mushroom Powder

The mushroom powder is a powder made from dried, crushed or ground edible mushrooms without any additional ingredients, which is used as a spice for soups and sauces.

For the production, mushrooms and mushroom remain, mostly of different types - as long as they are not corrupt or rotten - are first cut and dried until they are brittle and fragile. The pieces are then finely crushed in the mortar or mechanically ground into powder. The packaged airtight, mushroom powder will last for years. Unlike dried mushrooms, it does not need to be soaked or cooked for a long time to develop its aroma.

The commercially available mushroom powder may have a water content of at most 9 per cent by weight and an acid-insoluble ash content of not more than 3 per cent by weight according to the German food book.

Mushroom powder in capsules, like a pressed tablet or loose powder from so-called vital or medicinal mushrooms, are also offered on the European market as food supplements. The unprocessed mushrooms are dried and ground to powder. Special care is required here for allergy sufferers, since the powder may contain both "fungal spores, fungal dust, heat-sensitive hydrogen cyanide and polysaccharides and fungal toxins".

The mushroom powder can be stored very well and used for many applications. The production from a tough mushroom is more demanding than with soft mushrooms (which are very easy).

In principle, the mushroom must be prepared so that it is in small pieces or, better still, coarse powder (see "Shredding").

The following has proven itself for medicinal mushroom powder production:

- A coffee grinder or spice grinder
- Slow-running grain mills (high-speed "burn" the mushroom)
- Kitchen mixer with proper knives and a powerful motor
- Hand rubbing or electric rubbing with a fine friction blade

In principle, all mushrooms that are also suitable for drying are ideal for pulverizing. Here is a list:

- Acker parasol mushroom
- Anischampignons
- Lycoperdon pyriforme
- Birch mushrooms
- Bohemian Verpel
- Boletus aureus
- Butter mushrooms
- Real Mousseron
- Pea scatterer (Bohemian truffle)
- Gold-stemmed achievement
- Hasenohr
- Rabbit Boletus (Cinnamon Boletus)
- Hasenstäubling
- Herkuleskeule
- Maroon mugging
- Granule Boletus (Loachling)
- Coral mushrooms (all edible)
- Frizzy mother hen (fat hen)
- Bay boletes
- Morel cup Ling

- Morels
- Fairy Ring Mushroom
- Parasol mushrooms (stems)
- Knights (all edible)
- Rotkappen
- Crimson Ink (Stems)
- Pig's ear
- Ceps
- Stockschwämmchen
- Dead Trumpet (Autumn Trumpet)
- Trompetenpfifferling
- Truffles
- Worm-shaped club
- Scutage pes-caprae
- Goat's lips

Grind

A hand mill is sufficient for grinding. My beloved Zassenhaus grain mill has been serving me faithfully and impartially for about 25 years. The robust grinder of this classic is infinitely adjustable according to coarse or elegant; so many types of mushrooms and cereals have beeb ground over the decades.

If you like it electric or have ambitions towards a permanently operated grain grinder, we recommend the Fidibus 21 (250 watts) or the Fidibus Medium (360 watts) from Komo.

Store mushroom powder

The powder must be stored in dark glass jars that can be closed quickly (pharmacy jars). They are labelled with the respective type and should be fresh and dry.

Use of the powder

With powdered mushrooms, soups, sauces and broths can not only be seasoned and seasoned. They can also be made exclusively from powder, especially if they are to be beautiful or festive. The food in itself then "carries" the soup or sauce; everything else is an addition.

Mushroom cream sauce with mushroom powder for 4–6 people.

Ingredients

- 5-10 grams of the finest or 25 grams of coarse mushroom powder
- Freshly ground black pepper
- One full MSP salt
- 2 tbsp. butter
- Two tablespoons of shallots soaked in oil
- 200 ml. white wine
- 300 ml. cream (cream)
- 4 tbsp. finely chopped parsley

Preparation

1. Put the mushroom powder, pepper and salt in the melted butter in the boiling frying pan.
2. To sear STH. Put deglaze and shallots with the white wine. Add the cream.
3. Simmer the sauce to the desired consistency (thickness).
4. Mix in the parsley.
5. Ready-fried mushrooms can be added to the sauce as desired.

A schnitzel or a piece of meat is well suited to be smeared with an oil that is aromatically related to the mushroom - such as walnut, argan or truffle oil - and sprinkled sparingly with mushroom powder. Let it steep overnight. Prepared the next day, you will look forward to a highly exquisite dining experience. Mushroom powder in the highest dosage is also suitable for salads.

Alcoholic Mushroom Extract: Tincture

Tinctures have been used since ancient times as a way of preserving and utilizing the valuable ingredients of various medicinal plants. These concentrated plant extracts, mushroom extracts, elixirs and essences have always been used as natural medicines. Some of them are legendary, Paracelsus believed in the 16th century to have found a panacea in the opium tincture known as "laudanum".

Tinctures still play an essential role in medicine today. The alcoholic plant extracts are rich in natural essential oils, antioxidants, anti-inflammatory, antibacterial and antiviral substances and sometimes even cancer-inhibiting materials, they allow the active substances to be extracted efficiently and at the same time easily and mostly from mushroom. The removal of the heating elements with a solvent in alcohol is called maceration, and the resulting tinctures are also called macerates.

Tinctures Are Versatile

The concentrated plant extracts can be used in a variety of ways for health and personal care, as a replacement for numerous conventional medicines and also in nutrition. Most are probably best aware of cough drops or gastric drops, in which tinctures of individual plants are used undiluted. Tinctures can also be used as an ingredient in numerous natural cosmetics and care products such as homemade creams, lotions, toothpaste or shampoo and hair lotions.

Also, they are a gentle and particularly environmentally friendly alternative to essential oils, the increased use of which is particularly problematic for water bodies and which are considered to be environmentally hazardous and toxic to aquatic organisms in larger quantities.

These are enough reasons to make and use the valuable essences yourself!

What Is Needed

Fresh or dried herbs or other parts of plants are required as the starting material for homemade tinctures. However, they should no longer be too damp or even wet.

Almost all neutral types of alcohol are suitable as solvents, e.g. highly concentrated wine spirit (available in the pharmacy or online), Primasprit mixed alcohol as well as single grain or vodka with at least 40% alcohol by volume. When using new parts of the plant, the higher alcohol content is recommended because the water content of the plants slightly reduces the total alcohol content.

If you want to avoid alcohol as a solvent for various reasons, you can still use homemade tinctures. In a very similar way, alcohol-free tinctures can be produced using vinegar extract!

This is needed to make your alcoholic tinctures:

- 50 g. dried or 100 g. fresh herbs, cleaned and crushed
- 200 ml. of alcohol
- Screwed glass for ripening, e.g. an empty jam jar
- Coffee filter to filter the finished tincture
- Brown glass dropper bottles for storage

Home Made Tinctures

The process is easy but needs a few perseverances. Pour 50 g. of dried or 100 g. of fresh plant parts into a screw-top jar and pour in 200 ml. of alcohol. All parts of the plant should be covered entirely. Close the jar tightly, and it must now ripen for at least four weeks. Of course, you can vary the amounts in the same mixing ratio.

During this time, the alcohol gradually dissolves the soluble ingredients from the plants, which can be recognized by the colour that is created. You can help the process by gently shaking the jar once a day. Setting up in a warm and sunny place also speeds up the extraction. However, light-sensitive components can be damaged.

After the maturation period, the finished tinctures are poured through a beautiful coffee filter and filled into dropper bottles made of brown glass or other dark containers. You are now ready to use - don't forget to label the bottles right away!

Different Tinctures and Possible Uses

In principle, finished tinctures contain a large part of the active ingredients of their original plants in a concentrated form. Under here, you will get some approaches for possible ingredients and the potential uses of the tinctures.

Daisy tincture from the flower heads helps against blemished skin, blackheads and acne, it is dabbed on with a cosmetic pad or cotton ball and has a skin-clarifying and anti-inflammatory effect.

A comfrey tincture can be used internally and externally for all types of injuries and pain; it has an analgesic, anti-inflammatory, wound healing and cooling effect.

Typical cold herbs such as mint, thyme, sage, chamomile or elderflower are ideal for cough drops.

Chestnut tincture helps with skin problems such as acne, eczema and wounds, serves as the basis for homemade venous angel, it strengthens the blood vessels, promotes blood circulation and relieves varicose veins. It also supports rheumatism, joint pain and haemorrhoids.

A natural sedative and sleeping pill can be made from valerian roots using a tincture.

A carnation tincture is ideal for toothache and as an addition to homemade dental care products. It also helps with flatulence and is used to treat insect bites.

Just like cloves, clove root can also be used for tinctures to strengthen the gums.

Tinctures from celandine, thuja (tree of life, can only be used externally due to its toxicity), dandelions or garlic are used for the gentle treatment of warts.

Bedstraw can be used in the form of a tincture to strengthen the immune system, especially as a preventive cure in preparation for the cold season.

A tincture of the cowslip is suitable as a balm for nerve pain and fungal infections, internally it supports coughs, migraines, headaches, rheumatism and gout.

These are only a few samples of how homemade tinctures can help naturally, replacing numerous medications or reducing their need.

Here you can find more uses for tinctures:

- Ginger tincture for headache, nausea and colds
- Dandelion root tincture strengthens the spirits and cleanses the joints
- Root tincture against tight muscles
- Wild herb tincture for muscle pain
- Wild herb tincture as a natural headache remedy
- Homemade St. John's wort tincture

- Chestnut blossom tincture to strengthen the blood vessels and cough
- Athlete's tincture
- Tincture with horseradish and nasturtium as a natural antibiotic
- Alleviate mosquito bites with plantain tincture
- Homemade yarrow tincture as a natural helper for inflammation, bleeding and much more
- Red clover tincture - a natural helper for women suffering from colds and more
- Lavender tincture for sleep problems, migraines and much more
- Marigold tincture - natural help for inflammation, nausea and wounds
- Homemade stone clover tincture for heavy legs, migraines and much more
- Field horsetail tincture - help with cystitis, acne, cellulite and much more
- You can find a lot more recipe ideas for tinctures and homemade care products in our book tips:

- Do you have a favourite tincture, how do you prepare it and how is it used?

External Use of Tinctures

A tincture for rubbing in, brushing, spraying or as a pad should not contain more than 25% alcohol. If necessary, they can be diluted with water. In the case of thicker tinctures or sensitive skin conditions, it is advisable to cover neighbouring areas of the skin with a fatty ointment before use. After use, the surface should always be treated with a good cream (e.g. marigold), because alcohol dries out the skin.

For rinsing and gargling, a tincture is diluted 1:10 with water (10 to 20 drops of tincture per right sip of water). Gargle or rinse your mouth intensely for several minutes ("pull through your teeth"). The gargled water should not be swallowed.

Tinctures can be used as a base for room sprays. To make sprays more intense, add a few drops of essential oils. With remaining tinctures, you can also prepare an herbal bath (guide value: 5 to 10 tablespoons for a full bathroom).

On the subject of healing with tinctures, I would like to refer to the book Healing with Fresh Plant Drops by Bruno Vonarburg.

Dry Mushroom Tee

As you've already read, drying mushrooms is the best way to keep them. Some cooks even prefer dried mushrooms (porcini, morels, shiitake) to fresh mushrooms for sauces because they are more aromatic. Before using dried mushrooms are soaked in lukewarm water for about 30 minutes (for morels only 5 min), depending on the volume of the mushroom slices, so that the mushrooms can absorb the extracted water again.

Occasionally it would be best if you shook them to loosen the sand. After swelling, the mushrooms are to be used like fresh mushrooms. Warning: Don't pour the water in which you put the mushroom to increase, pour it through a sieve and use it to infuse your dish. This spring water contains so many mushroom aromas that give your meal even more taste. How much per person? 30 grams of dried mushrooms correspond to 250 to 300 grams of fresh mushrooms. You need about 10 to 15 grams and 1/4 litre of water per person to soak.

Mushroom Recipe

I am not a gourmet cook. Although I have lived alone since the age of 18, I am therefore able to prepare my food myself and it is also somewhat tasty (at least that is how I feel). With the creation of new recipes, however, I have hardly spent my previous life. Therefore, I hope that readers of the site will help here with recipes from their pool and allow me to publish them here under their name. From me only a relatively sparse beginning, it's a kind of coincidence when experimenting with the spice rack: since in the season I usually only get to use dry mushrooms or at most, a "recipe" with dried mushrooms.

Steinpilz-Crostini

Recipe by Katharina Krieglsteiner
Ingredients:

- One baguette
- 400 g. porcini mushrooms
- Two cloves of garlic (one finely chopped, the other whole)
- One small chilli pepper (finely chopped)

- 2 tbsp. marjoram
- 12 tbsp. olive oil
- Salt, pepper

Preparation:

1) Rinse the porcini mushrooms and slice them into thin wedges.
2) Cut two baguettes into slices and roast in the oven at 225 ° C until the slices are crispy.
3) Meanwhile, fry the finely chopped garlic and the chopped chilis in 6 tablespoons of olive oil, add the mushrooms before the garlic gets colored.
4) Add the marjoram after about 5 minutes and season with salt and pepper.
5) Rub the toasted bread with the clove of garlic and drizzle the remaining olive oil on it.
6) Now put the fried mushrooms on top and serve immediately.

Pickled Stimulants

Recipe by Katharina Krieglsteiner

Ingredients:

- 500 g. stimulus core (spruce, salmon or noble stimulus core)

For the brew:
- 125 ml. of vinegar
- 250 ml. of water
- Two bay leaves
- One sprig of rosemary
- One sprig of thyme
- Two cloves of garlic
- About ten whole peppercorns
- One tablespoon of sugar
- Salt
- Olive oil

Preparation:

1) Thoroughly rinse the mushrooms and cut them into pieces.
2) Simmer the peeled and halved garlic together with the remaining brewing ingredients on a low flame for 15 minutes.
3) In the meantime, boil the mushrooms in salted water for about 8 minutes, then drain and rinse. Then simmer in the broth for 5 minutes.

4) Put the mushrooms warm in carefully cleaned glasses, pour a portion of the food over each and top up with olive oil.

5) Close the jars well and let them go through for at least two weeks.

Pea Streaking Vegetables

A lovely load of vegetables - preferably varieties with a taste that is not too intense, e.g. Zucchini, Chinese cabbage, eggplants, etc. Prepare as usual with cream sauce and season with salt, omit other (intense) spices. To do this (while making) grate a slice of dried pea sprinkler into the dish. A poem! The pea spreader (Pisolithus Aarhus) is also called "slate truffle" in Germany. Katharina and I were able to collect and dry a fair amount of them in various places in the Portuguese Alentejo in December. The mushrooms - especially dried - have an incomparable, mushroom-like aroma and give every dish an exceptional note.

Dried Witch Boletus in Allspice Sauce

Please take a good handful or more dried slices of witch bolete (Boletus erythropus) and soak them in plenty of water for about 2 hours.

Add a teaspoon (or 2) full of allspice powder (sooner or later). Also, vegetable broth and salt, then bring to the boil and let it steep for a while. Add different amounts of cream, depending on your taste. The whole thing goes with pasta (e.g. ribbon pasta), but also with all other side dishes (i.e. potatoes, rice).

Some Interesting Facts

A gastronomic delicacy par excellence in autumn and winter, mushrooms also stand out for their dietary value to control weight. And beyond the flavors and food, they are also related to numerous aspects of our popular culture - there are mobile applications to help go out to look for mushrooms in the mountains - and they are even ancestral with our ancient religions. On the other hand, they move in an economic sector that although it is very seasonal, is not negligible: it is estimated that 200 million Euros are moved in Spain each year around the mushroom business.

Since November is the month of mushrooms, especially if October has been rainy and warm, as has happened this year, we explain ten curiosities that you have ignored about the world of fungi and mushrooms in case you dare to enter this world. You are fond of going out to the mountains on Saturdays for mushrooms instead of going to look at the Rolex of the corner jewellery.

Plants or Animals?

Mushrooms are the outer part of some fungi that live underground or within decaying organic matter. There are, however, many types of fungus, because they are one of the five kingdoms in which we group living beings and, therefore, are not considered plants or animals. They do not perform photosynthesis like vegetables, nor are they capable of eating as we do in the animal kingdom.

In the kingdom of fungi, they are from those who live in our intestinal flora to yeasts that ferment flour, vine or barley, through mold or those that attack the soles of our feet. And of course, also those who take mushrooms.

Why Do Mushrooms Exist in the World?

Especially mushrooms that make mushrooms are characterized by living underground or in decomposing organic matter. Their job is to absorb the results of such decomposition to feed, and they can also collect minerals from the soil. These fungi, which are large networks of cell filaments arranged as if they were connected train cars (mycelium), can pass crystals from one cell to another cell along each of the threads (hyphae).

On the other hand, many of them are connected to the roots of the trees in a mixed organ called mycorrhiza. This organ is symbiotic; that is, it is a collaborative centre of both beings. It allows the tree to contribute sugars to the fungus and the fungus to bring minerals from remote sites for the tree through its filaments. Also, a fungus can be connected to several trees and even an entire forest, thus forming a kind of organic Internet for that forest.

Well, in the state of Oregon, in the North Pacific of the United States, a single fungus has been found that connects a 900-hectare forest, thus constituting the most massive known living being on the planet. It is suspected that such interconnected fungi may also move antibiotic substances from a tree apart from different types of information, so it could be said that they are the intelligence of the forest.

Mushroom Is the Genitals of the Fungus

The mushroom is the gonads of the fungus, the organ that produces the spores through which the fungus mixes its genetic material. If you want, it can also be called the mushroom flower. Under the hat of the fungus, we can see some radial plates known as ' lamellae ', which are the producers of the spores that then disseminate the wind or the animals. The mushroom only manufactures the fungus after a period of rains, because it has enough moisture to create these hydraulic structures that are 90% water.

How Many Mushrooms Are Edible?

Only 0.001% of mushrooms are edible. There is a joke among mycologists - mushroom scholars - who say: "All mushrooms can be eaten, but most only once". In fact, of the 600,000 species of existing mushrooms, only 600 are known as edibles. The rest have different levels of toxicity due to the alkaloids they generate to protect themselves precisely from an animal attack, and some are directly moral. On the other hand, not all beings resist the same: the slug, for example, is 1,000 times more resistant than we are to the toxicity of mushrooms.

What Are Truffles?

Truffles are underground mushrooms. Truffles, both white (Tuber magnatum and black (Tuber melanosporum) are tuberous formations of spores of a fungus that forms mycorrhizae with chestnut, walnut, holm oak and oak trees of Southern Europe (Italy, France, Spain) and that grow under the ground instead of surfacing.

Mushroom Forests Are Already Cultivated

For more than twenty years the roots of freshly sprouted trees have been sprayed with spores of various fungi so that a mycorrhiza forms. Then they are planted in a field waiting for both the tree and the fungus to develop, and the latter ends up pulling mushrooms after the rainy season, which may take about five years to happen. Also, the most modern techniques allow spraying the seeds on a tree directly before planting it.

Can mushrooms be grown at home?

Yes, some mushrooms can be grown at home. Saprophytic fungi, decomposers of organic matter, such as mushrooms or oyster mushrooms, can be grown in a house if we have a dark, moist and cold area to let them work. A mixture of straw and feces from cattle that has been disinfected with fungus spores is used and packed. These packages are already sold commercially, and we have to store and water them periodically. Gradually mushroom mushrooms will appear on the surface.

Some Mushrooms Walk

The myxomycetes are a very peculiar group of fungi that form a sort of mass of clay instead of underground filaments. They live by decomposing organic matter, especially logwood in humid forests and have bright yellow, red or orange colours. They appear as a melted candle or a mass of plasticine and move to find material to decompose. They do this thanks to the creation of cellular plasma currents that are pushing the fungus in a specific direction.

Mushrooms Are the Traditional Religious Drug of Europe

The relationship between mushrooms and witchcraft is long and rich since some toxic mushrooms do not kill, but do have an intoxicating or hallucinogenic effect that served in the ancient liturgies of the witches. As a paradigm of this are the witch hoops, which are circles of mushrooms that appear in the forest clearings and are technically called 'arils'.

An 'aryl' is how the fungus usually removes all its string of mushrooms from a season and has a round shape to emit the spores in all directions better. They cannot always be seen complete, but in medieval Europe, when they saw each other, it was believed that the devil lived in its center.

On the other hand, the dwarfs in the stories inhabit red hat mushrooms with white tips because this species of mushroom, Amanita muscaria, is hallucinogenic and who ate it, saw people deformed in their hallucinations. It is also believed that there is an intimate relationship between mystics such as Santa Teresa and San Juan de la Cruz and a fungus called 'ergot of rye', which affected rye bread and caused hallucinations to those who ate it.

It is also believed that El Greco was fond of hallucinogenic mushrooms, as well as Antoni Gaudí. Hence, according to this theory, their peculiar aesthetic conceptions would start, with elongated shapes, bright colours and many curves in their geometry.

Why Are They Picked up with Wicker Baskets?

The wicker basket used by the collectors has an ecological right: to help the fungus to expand. When we put the mushroom in the basket, it is loose spores that with our movement through the forest are falling to the ground through the gaps left by the wicker braid, so that we are distributing them.

How to Cure Depression and Stress

Depression treatment through psilocybin-assisted psychotherapy is being examined. Two other studies investigate the possibility that psilocybin can alleviate the psychological suffering associated with cancer. A study, conducted by Charles Grob, involves 12 people with terminal cancer who were given hallucinogen or placebos in two separate sessions. The second study, conducted by Roland Griffiths, administered psilocybin to people who "with a diagnosis of cancer who have some anxiety or feel depressed about their condition".

First results indicated that low doses of psilocybin can improve mood and reduce patients' anxiety in advanced stages of the disease. These effects last from two weeks to six months. In the year 2008, a research team from the Johns Hopkins School of Medicine published guidelines for the responsible management of medical trials with psilocybin and other hallucinogens in humans.

Also, psilocybin has shown promise in relieving pain caused by cluster headaches, sometimes considered not one of the most painful problems, but as "one of the worst pains caused by syndromes known for humanity". In 2006, 22 of 26 cluster headache patients reported success in preventing attacks through the use of psilocybin, and 18 of 19 psilocybin users reported having more extended periods without suffering attacks.

How to Safely Heal Your Body

Preparation

When consuming mushrooms, you must keep in mind the following aspects related to their consumption: The set and setting conditions must be adequate for the excellent development of the fungal experience and avoid especially bad trips and accidents.

Set (the environment): it must be pleasant, friendly and safe.

Setting (mood): The person mustn't be going through a wrong personal time and must live the experience with a positive attitude.

The good concurrence of these two elements will allow the user to get carried away on the trip having an experience as pleasant and complete as possible. To avoid vomiting, it is convenient not to consume it with a full stomach and do it when the digestion is over.

Some Things to Consider

- Do not insist that someone consume or stop eating mushrooms, and this is a decision that everyone should make for himself. If someone does not want to waste it, it is better to respect that. Furthermore, remember that the company of someone sober is always good in case problems arise.
- Choose companions well, especially the first few times it is better to know and get along with who will be with us.
- If for something, there are bad rolls, better leave the consumption for another time.
- Choose the place well, consume in a place where you feel comfortable, safe and comfortable.
- Choose the moment well, avoid consuming if you are not on your best day.
- Calculate the dose well: if you plan to consume while partying and dancing, low or medium doses will be the most appropriate.
- High doses are best consumed in quiet contexts like a house. Due to the distinction in the scope of the mushrooms, it is best to measure the dosage in grams and not in the number of copies.

- Due to the variation in the content of psilocybin and psilocin between mushrooms and others, it is best to spray them so that we obtain a homogeneous concentration that will be the average of all the mushrooms we have.
- While the effects last, do not conduct or do activities that themselves may pose dangers or that require a good attention span and reflexes. Keep prudence until the end of the experience.
- Sometimes, the risks increase at the time of the descent, when there is a sense of "false security" that can lead us to carry out risky behaviors when we are not yet fully owners of ourselves.
- Before consumption, leave everything well tied and make sure you have no worries like having to return home at a specific time or similar things; especially with high doses. It can condition all experience preventing you from enjoying the desired effects and enhancing feelings of distress and loss of control.
- Also, keep in mind the next day when it comes to hangovers and downturns: make sure you have a quiet day, avoid problems, and let the experience rest and assimilate with pleasure.
- Try to consume on an empty stomach, at least a couple of hours without having eaten, thus

reducing possible stomach discomfort and making it easier to obtain more significant effects with lower doses.

- Eating some food (yoghurts, chocolate) at the end of the trip will produce pleasant sensations as well as help to recover nutrients and energies and will favor the taking of contact with reality.
- Be cautious with mixtures, especially with alcohol and amphetamines, and the stomach may suffer.

Psilocybin has transparently investigated as an experimental treatment for many diseases. In 1961, Timothy Leary and Richard Alpert carried out the Harvard Psilocybin Project, carrying out several experiments regarding the use of psilocybin in the treatment of personality disorders and other applications in psychological therapies.

A pilot study conducted by Francisco Moreno at the University of Arizona and funded by the Multidisciplinary Association for Psychedelic Studies examined the effects of psilocybin in nine patients with obsessive-compulsive disorder (OCD). He found that psilocybin can be safely administered to patients with OCD, resulting in a substantial reduction of its symptoms in many of the patients.

Herbal Benefits

The mushrooms are fantastic. They are not plants or animals but have an independent kingdom. Evolutionarily they are closer to animals, giving them new properties. They do not perform photosynthesis like plants, but they feed on dead matter, being the recyclers par excellence of nature.

They have been used for years in the East as medicine, and also as an essential element in their kitchen. Today you will know the secrets of these strange lifeforms and some ideas to take advantage of their healing capacity.

Mushrooms and Mycelia

Although we talk about mushrooms and truffles to refer to the same thing, they are different things. Mushrooms are the fruit of the fungus, whose main body remains hidden under the ground, forming an extensive network of filaments called mycelium.

In the words of the renowned mycologist Paul Stamets "the mycelium is the neurological network of nature", by orchestrating complex chemical and enzymatic responses to different requirements, from decomposing organic matter to producing defenses against bacteria. Fungi are the basis of many antibiotics, penicillin representing the fungus to which more people owe their lives. His discovery was a powerful weapon against the infectious diseases that decimated us.

The mycelium is also connected to the roots of plants and trees, exchanging nutrients with both, but also information. The plants themselves communicate with each other through this network, alerting, for example, the presence of certain parasites. For some, the mycelium is the Internet of nature.

Mushroom Benefits

Fungi are small pharmaceuticals. More than one hundred possible therapeutic effects of mushrooms are known, and many current drugs are based on medicinal mushrooms. For brevity, I will focus on the main benefits.

Nutritional Power

For starters, mushrooms have a high nutritional profile. They are rich in vitamin C and multiple vitamins of group B (especially niacin and riboflavin), in addition to providing minerals.

Since it's not vegetable nor animal, its protein has intermediate properties, surpassing the protein of cereals or legumes in biological value (except soybeans). Lots of mushrooms also provide all the essential amino acids.

Several fungi have a texture and flavor similar to meat, making them a suitable replacement in vegetarian diets.

Like us, mushrooms synthesize vitamin D when exposed to ultraviolet radiation, and although it is vitamin D_2, less effective than D_3, it is a very insignificant compliment.

Mushrooms are low in carbohydrates, being very attractive in ketogenic diets, and their fiber could contribute to improving the diversity of the microbiota.

Beyond the usual nutrients, they are a source of different compounds in other foods, such as different beta-glucans, a type of polysaccharide that gives many of the benefits that we will see below.

Improvement of the Immune System and Defense Against Bacteria

For starters, mushrooms provide compounds that directly help fight against different bacteria, and can even be used to treat resistant bacteria.

Multiple varieties exert an interesting modulating effect on the immune system that raises the production of our natural defenses.

In mice, supplementing the diet with mushrooms strengthens their adaptive immune system, improving survival against salmonella infection.

Some fungi, such as reishi, are considered adaptogens, and these regulate our stress response.

Anticancer Properties

Different anticancer drugs have their origin in fungi, by providing different bioactive compounds with an anticancer effect, which act through multiple mechanisms.

At the population level, the studies associate a higher consumption of mushrooms with a lower risk of different types of cancer.

Several compounds isolated from fungi have demonstrated effectiveness against cancer cells.

We are speaking about beta-glucans, and those present in mushrooms are especially potent in the fight against cancer. For example, lentinan is a beta-glucan present in the shiitake fungus, which increases survival and quality of life in cancer patients, and is used as a complement to conventional therapies.

Mental Health

Although there are few studies in humans, some mushrooms are associated with favorable effects at the cognitive level, in addition to helping to mitigate the symptoms of different neurodegenerative disorders.

The mushroom called Lion's Mane is especially useful in this regard for its contribution of an interesting bioactive molecule capable of crossing the blood-brain barrier and acting as a precursor to nerve growth factor. It would thus exercise its neuroprotective role, and even helps to reduce depression.

Weight Loss and Better Metabolic Health

Mushrooms are low in calories but highly satiating for their texture and high fiber intake. This combination is key to losing weight without starving.

In animals, extracts from different mushrooms reduce fat accumulation and improve the lipid profile.

At the metabolic level, they seem to improve fatty liver and glucose regulation, and also reduce low-grade inflammation that contributes to insulin resistance.

As we saw previously, mushrooms are in many areas closer to animals than to plants, and an example of this is their contribution of conjugated linoleic acid (LAC). This refreshing fatty acid could help control weight and improve metabolic health, among many other things. For example, people with more LAC in their bodies also have less risk of coronary heart disease.

Two important notes on conjugated linoleic acid:

- It is present in small amounts in meat and milk fat, especially in the case of grass-fed cows. Conventional meats and dairy hardly contribute to this compound.

- There are multiple different types (isomers) of LAC, and the versions used in supplements are generally different from those found in food. Although there are some favorable studies with supplements, most do not show any benefit, and their long-term effect is unknown. So, it is much better to obtain FTA from food.

Finally, the Maitake mushroom also provides a particular compound, called the SX fraction, that could combat the metabolic syndrome by reducing carbohydrate absorption.

Typical Mushrooms and Preparation Ideas

It is estimated that there are more than one million varieties of different mushrooms, most of them still unknown. Let's review below some of the most used and a few ideas to prepare them.

Common Mushroom

It is the most consumed mushroom in the world. Hence many times, talk about mushrooms and truffles interchangeably. However, truffles are simply a type of mushroom, the fruit of the fungus *Agaricus bisporus*.

Despite their conventional appearance, they are very nutritional. They contain more than 25% protein (dry), and much of their carbohydrate is beneficial fiber, including the famous beta-glucans. They also are rich in minerals.

You can eat them raw (for example, chopped on a salad), sautéed with vegetables, or scrambled with egg or cream.

The portobello is a variant of mushroom, and its larger size makes it very versatile in the kitchen. You can use them to replace the bread in a hamburger or add a raw egg and put them in the oven for a few minutes.

Shiitake

It is probably the second most popular mushroom. Although it is traditional Chinese cuisine, it is easily found in many supermarkets.

Its meat is dense and rich in iron, and also provides a particular amino acid: ergothioneine, which seems to protect our mitochondria. Some believe it could be a new vitamin with an important antioxidant and cytoprotective role.

Some of its compounds could also benefit oral health, by fighting, for example, caries causing bacteria.

You can prepare the shiitake as you want, but we like it, especially in risotto, also as part of vegetable soup.

Enoki

Another classic of Asian cuisine, and one of the first to be studied for its anticancer potential.

Dr. Tetsuro Ikekawa worked at the National Cancer Institute in Japan and wondered why cancer rates in Nagano Prefecture were unusually low compared to neighboring areas. When investigating, he discovered that Nagano was the center of cultivation of the enoki fungus, being especially appreciated among its inhabitants. Going deeper, he also observed that the families who cultivated these fungi developed less cancer than the rest of the population.

You can use them to prepare soups or stews, and also take advantage of their elongated shape to prepare them wrapped in bacon or ham.

Oyster Mushroom

It is rich in protein and vitamins B1, B2, and B3, in addition to providing new compounds that seem to improve mental health (study). It stimulates, for example, the nerve growth factor, and its effects are being studied when mitigating neurodegenerative diseases.

Although they usually grow on tree trunks, you can harvest them in your own home with a kit like this. For the first time, you'll be glad to see mushrooms growing in your kitchen.

Benefits of Eating Mushrooms

Your favorite season is autumn, and you love to pick mushrooms? In this book, we review all the benefits of eating mushrooms, backed by various scientific studies and with a long gastronomic tradition in ancestral cultures.

Races around the world have eaten and used mushrooms for medicinal purposes for centuries, since ancient Egypt. Legend has it that the pharaohs liked their earthy flavor so much that they declared fungi royalty food and forbade commoners to touch them. In Spain, some of the most consumed mushrooms are chanterelles, boletus, wild mushrooms or oronja mushrooms, although oyster or shiitake mushrooms are also consumed.

The eco-friendly material that will replace leather thanks to mushrooms.

In addition to weight loss and weight control, mushrooms stand out for their excellent nutritional value and the multiple benefits they provide to health. Today we review seven of them, taking advantage of the fact that we are at the ideal station for collection and consumption.

Anti-Cancer Properties

A research issued in the annual Experimental Biology and Medicine experimented five types of fungi - among which were oyster mushrooms or portobello mushrooms - and found that they "significantly suppressed" the growth and reproduction of breast cancer cells. It suggests that "common and special fungi may have a chemoprotective role against cancer of the breast". Also, shiitake lentinan is in mushrooms, a type of sugar molecule that helps extend the survival of patients with some types of cancer when used with chemotherapy. Japanese researchers studied more than 36,000 men for more than a decade and found that those who ate mushrooms three times or more per week had a 17% lower risk of developing prostate cancer.

Immune System Strength

Thanks to beta-glucan, a sugar that is found in the cell walls of fungi (among other plants) and also helps strengthen your immune system, mushrooms are ideal supplements that also help your heart.

Cholesterol Reduction

Since they are a good source of chitin and beta-glucan, they are cholesterol-lowering fibers. A study revealed the International Journal of Medicinal Mushrooms found that pink oyster mushrooms reduce total cholesterol and LDL ("bad" cholesterol) within hypercholesterolemic rodents. Shiitake mushrooms comprise a mixture that helps the liver process cholesterol and removes it from the bloodstream. Most mushrooms contain potent phytonutrients that help prevent cells from adhering to the walls of blood vessels, maintaining blood pressure and healthy circulation

Rich in Vitamins

Fungi are one of the few food sources for vitamin D, which our bodies can produce a fat-soluble vitamin that, with exposure to sunlight, and helps absorb calcium and promote bone growth. They are also rich in another vital vitamin: B12, which is crucial for vegetarians, since it's common frequently discovered in animal products, so mushrooms become a convincing meat substitute. This is not all since, in fungi, you will also find iron, phosphorus, iodine, magnesium, selenium, calcium, potassium, zinc, or vitamin A.

Anti-Inflammatory Powers

Fungi are rich in a powerful antioxidant called ergothioneine, which helps reduce inflammation throughout the body. Highlights include reishi mushrooms in particular, which have been used medicinally in Asia for thousands of years to fight disease, reduce inflammation, suppress allergic responses, etc.

Against the Aging

In a study published in Penn State, researchers discovered that fungi have large amounts of two antioxidants, ergothioneine, and glutathione, which are associated with anti-aging properties. Another 2019 study found that older people who ate 300 grams and more of roasted mushrooms a week were half as likely to have mild cognitive impairment. The six-year study, conducted between 2011 and 2017, collected data from more than 600 adults over 60 living in Singapore. Researchers said they analyzed ergothioneine as the possible reason for this impact.

The Various Strains of Psilocybin

The psilocybin toxicity is low; in rats, the average lethal dose is approximately 280 mg/kg, about 75% times more significant than that of caffeine. When administered intravenously in rabbits, the LD 50 of psilocybin is about 12.5 mg/kg (rabbits, however, are extremely intolerant of the effects of most psychoactive drug effects.

The deadly dose of psilocybin alone is unknown in the case of recreational or medicinal levels and has never been documented; a case reported in 2008 said: "Death due to ingestion of psilocybin alone is unknown for recreational or medicinal levels". Psilocybin at most corresponds to 1% of the total mushroom weight of *Psilocybe Cubensis*, and approximately 1.7 kilograms of evaporated mushrooms or 17 kilograms of fresh mushrooms would be needed for a 60 kg person to reach the LD 50 of 280 mg/kg measure for rats.

Psilocybin is absorbed through the mouth and stomach. The effects begin 10-40 minutes after ingestion of fungi containing psilocybin and lasts 2-6 hours depending on the dose, the species of the fungus and the metabolism of the individual. A typical recreational treatment is 10–50 mg of psilocybin. Nevertheless, a minimal amount of people remain unusually sensitive to the consequences of psilocybin, where a threshold dose of about 2 mg of psilocybin results in effects generally associated with medium to high doses. In the same way, some people require relatively high doses to achieve the typical impact of a small treatment.

Brain chemistry and the metabolism of the individual, play a significant role in the individual's response to psilocybin. Most of the psilocybin is metabolized in the liver where it is converted into psilocin, which is degraded by the monoamine oxidase enzyme to produce various metabolites in the blood plasma including 4-hydroxy indole-3-acetaldehyde, 4-hydroxytryptophan and 4-hydroxy indole -3-acetate.

Sometimes psilocybin is not enzymatically degraded and instead forms a glucuronide - a biochemical method used by animals to remove toxic substances by binding with a glucuronic acid, which is excreted in the urine. Plasma psilocin concentrations in adult volunteers average around 8μg / L within 2 hours after ingestion of a single oral dose of 15 mg of psilocybin; psychological effects occur with a plasma concentration of 4–6 μg / L.

Physical and mental tolerance to psilocybin occurs and dissipates rapidly. Ingestion of psilocybin more than three or four times in a week (especially on consecutive days) may decrease its effects. Tolerance is eliminated after a few days; frequent users intersperse doses in spaces of five to seven days to avoid this tolerance effect. Studies have shown that cross-tolerance can develop between psilocybin and the pharmacologically similar compound LSD. The monoamine oxidase (MAOI) sustains the effects of psilocybin for longer; therefore, people who take MAOI due to a medical problem may experience highly potentiated effects.

Consistently use of psilocybin does not lead to a physical dependence on the drug. A 2008 study concluded that, based on information from the United States for the period 2000-2002, in a group of adolescents (defined between 11-17 years of age) the use of hallucinogenic drugs (including psilocybin) does not increase the risk of drug dependence in adulthood; in contrast to the application during adolescence of cannabis, cocaine, inhalants, anxiolytic drugs and stimulants, which are all associated with "an increased risk of developing clinical features associated with drug dependence".

The Effects of Psilocybin

The American psychologist Timothy Leary performed the first experiments of the effects caused by psychedelic drugs, such as psilocybin.

The results of psilocybin are very variable and depend on the mentality and scenario in which the consumer is at during the time of experiencing such effects. It is commonly called a set and setting. In the early 1960s, Leary and his colleagues at Harvard University undertook experiments to understand the role of set and setting on the results of psilocybin. The drug was administered to 175 people from different social backgrounds in a warm and comfortable environment free from distractions; to make it similar to a quiet living room.

Ninety-eight of these people were given questionnaires to evaluate their experiences and the contribution of social and circumstantial factors. Those individuals who had already taken psilocybin described more pleasant experiences than those who had not. Group size, dose, preparation and expectations were essential determinants of the response to the drug. The large groups (of eight or more individuals) were described negatively as less encouraging by the members, and their experiences were less pleasant.

Conversely, the smaller groups (less than six) were seen more comprehensively, and those who made that group up showed positive reactions to the drug. The researchers proposed that psilocybin probably causes an increase in suggestibility, making the individual more receptive to interpersonal interactions or environmental stimuli. These conclusions were corroborated in a later study by Berge (1999), who concluded that: dose and set and setting are fundamental and definitive factors in experiments that tested the effects of psychedelic drugs on artists' creativity.

After the consumption of psilocybin, the person may initially feel somewhat disoriented, lethargic and euphoric or sometimes depressed. With low doses, hallucinatory effects can occur, such as the more intense perception of colours or the animation of geometric shapes. The hallucination with eyes closed may be experienced where the individual can see geometric shapes multi-colored and vivid imaginary series.

At higher doses, hallucinatory effects development and happenings lead to be limited social and more introspective or entheogenic. Hallucinations with open eyes are more common and can be very detailed, although they can rarely be confused with reality. Based on a knowledge of 27 hospital admissions of patients (aged 12-24 years) who had used *Psilocybe semilanceata*, a 1980 clinical record summed the division of clinical signs caused by psilocybin overdose such as the following:

- Perception disorder (23 patients)
- Mydriasis (pupil dilation) (20)
- Dysphoria (13)
- Hyperreflexia (12)
- Tachycardia (10)
- Lethargy (7)
- Euphoria (5)

These clinical responses are similar to the results obtained in several of the first studies where pure human psilocybin was administered to human volunteers.

Perception Disorder

Perception disorders are varied and may be due to different causes such as:

- Infections, tumors or other types of organic brain lesions
- Poisoning by alcohol, drugs or other substances
- Emotional or psychic causes

The primary disorders of perception are:

- Illusions of false impressions of a real external stimulus, that is, it is a misinterpretation of a typical foreign sensory experience.
- Hallucinations, which are false perceptions with the absence of an external stimulus, in other words, is the perception of a foreign object without such a purpose. It is because the subject attributes an internal psychological event to an external source.

- Hallucinations can be visual, auditory, olfactory, tactile, etc.
- Among the most frequent alterations of perception produced by organic causes, we will mention Agnosia, and among those caused by emotional reasons, we will point out the Macropsy.

<u>Mydriasis</u>

Mydriasis is controlled by the sympathetic nervous system, which causes contraction of the iris dilator muscle.

Mydriasis is a normal reaction to penumbra. In that case, it is bilateral and reactive; the lighting of one eye triggers the regression of the mydriasis of the two eyes. This reaction and its opposite require the integrity of a circuit that includes:

- Retina
- Optic nerve
- Brain areas of vision
- Pupil

Pupillary diameter dilation can be caused by some drugs, such as atropine, some toxic substances, substances of abuse, cocaine, and alcohol; and it can also be related to focused brain lesions, for example, of the brainstem, or it can be one of the reactions of the panic syndrome. It can be a symptom of a disease in some cases, or brain damage, such as in a cardiorespiratory arrest, but also certain comas of diverse origin.

It can also accompany some facial paralysis.

Mydriasis, in one or both eyes, is sometimes observed after surgery performed near the nerve or one of its branches and by complex fractures. It occurs relatively frequently after dental interventions in caries treatments, in which case it usually affects only one of the eyes.

The trigeminal nerve lesion, which controls various parts of the face, is usually irreversible, with the pupil permanently dilated. Sensitivity is provided by the trigeminal nerve or V cranial nerve. Trigeminal nerve lesions produce various symptoms, from paralysis to jaw pain or migraines such as trigeminal neuralgia or Claude-Bernard-Horner syndrome. The blink that occurs the corneal reflex is when the cornea is touched, the afferent pathway goes through the trigeminal nerve and the flickering response, through the facial nerve.

Mydriatic agents are substances that induce pupil dilation, for example, atropine, tropicamide, or

Dubois in sulfate. They act in different ways, such as cocaine, for example, inhibits the reabsorption of norepinephrine at the neuromuscular synapse. When it is stated that a solution of cocaine affects the eye, it is because norepinephrine is no longer reabsorbed by neurons, and increases its levels.

Norepinephrine is a neurotransmitter of the central nervous system and causes such pupil dilation. Artificial mydriasis can be performed by the instillation of eye drops with atropine in the eye. This is mostly used for specific ophthalmological exams, such as observation of the fundus.

In symmetric is active mydriasis, the two pupils dilate and do not contract in the light, which is a sign of significant brain damage, as can be seen in cardiorespiratory arrest, but also specific comas.

It is usually easily differentiated from myosis, in which a pupil would be more contracted since the dilated pupil is much more contracted than it should with normal stimuli. It often does not react by contracting at all. The observation of the pupils and the test of the pupillary reflexes are part of the evaluation of the neurological state of a patient.

Dysphoria

The dysphoria is generally characterized as an unpleasant or uncomfortable emotion, such as sadness (depressed mood), anxiety, irritability or restlessness. It is the etymological opposite of euphoria.

Dysphoria refers only to a disorder of emotions and can be experienced in response to ordinary life events, such as illness or grief. Also, it is a feature of many psychiatric disorders, such as anxiety disorders and mood disorders. Dysphoria is usually experienced during depressive episodes, but people with bipolar disorder may also experience it during manic or hypomanic episodes. Dysphoria, in the context of an emotional disorder, is an indicator of the high risk of suicide.

Dysphoria can be chemically induced by agonist substances of the opioid kappa receptor. Dysphoria is also one of the symptoms of hypoglycemia.

It also occurs in cases of transsexuality, commonly called gender dysphoria. Being discussed, even if they are pathologies, dysphoria is present because of the conditions and situations to which these people are exposed.

The ability of Xéneru and the term col qu'n in 1973 the doctor John Money, and from the beginning of psychiatry, designate what in 1953 the doctor also Harry Benjamin will call transsexual date.

The DSM IV or Diagnostic and Statistical Manual of the mental disorders appears to be the name of the sexual identity. As of DSM-5, it is recategorized as xéneru dysphoria. Nel ICD-10 continues to be called restoring d'identidá de xéneru.

There are two components to the condition that has to take into account the diagnosis. First of all, you have conclusive evidence that the individual identifies, reliably and persistently, col otru sexu, which constituted the desire to be, or the insistence that it belonged to the other person to whom it was assigned.

Secondly, if you also need to try persistent discomfort, you may experience a feeling of inadequacy along the lines of sex or gender. To diagnose Xéneru's, dysphoria has evidence of clinically significant distress or social deterioration, labor, or other essential areas of the individual's life. It is of the utmost importance to refute children and adolescents where their behavior does not fit into the cultural stereotype of masculinity or femininity.

Nowadays, there is not a method to diagnose it because it depends purely on what the effect or what manifests, so the occasions are biased with or without intentionality.

On the other hand, according to a report by the American Foundation for Suicide Prevention and the Williams Institute, suicide attempts can reach 41%, compared to the 5% that the non-Tresxéneru population re-registers, being more significant cases of people who submit or they wanted to undergo ciruís de cambéu de sexu. The authors of the report repaired an interrelation between stress factors (such as experiences of discrimination and ill-treatment) and three types of mental health that raises a particular vulnerability to suicide among the three-person or non-conforming person.

Gender dysphoria is the same as an intersexual physical illness after the first have normal genitalia in contrast to ambiguous genital colic or hypogonadism find in intersexual physical diseases, such as androgen insensitivity syndrome or hyperplasia congenital adrenal. Its causes are still unknown, although biological, psychological, and even sociological hypotheses have been taken into consideration. From the non-medical explanations, many sectors require it to be considered a psychiatric disorder.

Hyperreflexia

In medicine, it is known as hyperreflexia to the exaltation or increase of the osteotendinous reflexes, and it is, therefore, the opposite phenomenon to the decrease of hyporeflexia. Hyperreflexia is detected by the doctor during clinical examination, usually using the reflex hammer and exploring the patellar reflex, percussion in the homonymous tendon. It was also diagnosed by examining other reflexes, including the Aquilian reflex, bicipital reflex, tricipital reflex, radial style reflex, and cubitopronator reflex. Various diseases can cause it, and one of the most frequent is the pyramidal lesion.

The causes can be varied; one of the most frequent is the pyramidal lesion, which can be affected by numerous neurological diseases. Some of the most common are:

Cerebral palsy.

- Cerebral hemorrhage
- Cerebral embolism
- Transient ischemic attack
- Brain tumor
- Meningitis

- Multiple sclerosis
- Spinal cord injury
- Amyotrophic lateral sclerosis

Other causes of hyperreflexia include hyperthyroidism, electrolyte disturbances, serotonin syndrome, Reyes syndrome, and intoxication by certain drugs of abuse.

Tachycardia

The tachycardia is the increase (acceleration) of the heartrate. It happens when the ventricles contract too fast. It is considered when the heartrate is higher than 100 beats per minute at rest.

It can be physiological (that is, not pathological), for example, when intense physical activity is performed or when intense emotions occur (fear, anxiety, worries, nervousness about some everyday situation, or any other feeling derived from stress). It can also be associated with pathological processes, such as anemia, hemorrhages, insomnia or not sleeping correctly, shock, kidney failure, depression, the infection of some organs, excessive nervousness, and others.

Tachycardia alone does not affect life expectancy significantly. This symptom is more common in women than in men. It can be caused by factors such as smoking, alcoholism, drugs, or deficiency of the thyroid gland. It also varies depending on emotions, pain, and thoughts.

An electrocardiogram (the recording of the electrical activity of the heart) makes it possible to detect possible arrhythmias. In some cases, it is necessary to resort to the placement of a Holter monitor, a device that is attached to the patient's body and allows recording the electrical activity of the heart.

The heart acts as a pump that drives blood circulation throughout the body. The muscle fibers of the heart must contract in unison to function as expected. Bioelectric impulses from a group of cells located in the right atrium govern the contractions of the heart; These impulses flow along paths that communicate with the muscle fibers of the four chambers.

When any part of this complex conduction system is damaged, the regular rhythm of the heartbeat is disturbed. As a result, different heart disorders can occur, such as cardiac arrest, ventricular fibrillation, atrial fibrillation, heart block, or tachycardia, but the patient must be 12 years old or older to get this disease. According to statistics, 98 percent of children with this problem die as adults, between 41 and 53 years of age.

Causes of Tachycardia

The tachycardia is more common in women than in men. And maybe due to different reasons:

- Arterial hypertension
- Heart disease
- Coronary heart disease
- Infections
- Lung diseases
- Renal insufficiency
- Stress
- Alcohol or drug abuse
- Smoking
- Caffeine Abuse
- Strong emotions
- Excessive intake of caffeine

Symptoms of Tachycardia

Tachycardia includes the appearance of specific symptoms, such as:

- Dizziness
- Choking sensation or respiratory distress
- Sudden weakness
- Trembling in the chest
- Vertigo
- Syncope.

Tachycardia may occur sporadically or occasionally, but frequently, it may be a symptom of severe disease such as arrhythmia and therefore, if you have it you should consult with the doctor so they can set the appropriate diagnosis and treatment.

Lethargy

Lethargy is a state of prolonged drowsiness caused by certain diseases. It is also a symptom of several nervous, infectious, or toxic diseases, characterized by a state of deep and prolonged sleepiness. Clumsiness, drowsiness, callousness, alienation of mood-related to this state as associated behaviors since our organism relaxes our entire body.

It is a clinical picture related to fatigue or asthenia and, in severe cases, to narcolepsy. It is also considered a particular type of hibernation characteristic of some alpine mammals in polar areas, such as the groundhog, the bear, the lirón, the recently found Patagonian Berni, etc.

Lethargy is the temporary or complete loss of sensibility and movement due to unknown physiological causes, leading the individual into a morbid state in which vital functions are attenuated. The lifeform appears to be suspended, giving the body the appearance of death.

The patient lies motionless, the limbs hanging without any stiffness, breathing and pulse are almost invisible, and the pupils dilated and unresponsive to light. There are cases where the patient, despite absolute inertia, perceives and understands everything, but is unable to react at all. Because of the mental activity conserved during this lethargic state, it is called lucid lethargy.

In the past, due to the lack of medical resources, there were cases of people reported as dead. Subsequently, in the case of exhumations, it was found that the corpse was in a different position from the one in which it was placed in the coffin or scratched lids, suggesting that such people were buried alive during a lethargic state. Currently, medicine recognizes death as only people who do not have any brain activity, which would make such an event impossible. Watching the movie "Awakening Time" gives you a clear idea of an example of lethargy

Euphoria

Euphoria is medically recognized as a state of mind and emotions in which a person experiences intense feelings of well-being, happiness, excitement, and joy. Technically, euphoria can be considered an affect, but colloquially it is used to define emotion as a heightened state of transcendent happiness with an immense sense of satisfaction.

The most popular use of the theory, though, is connected with the sense of well-being. The euphoria can range from gratitude to glorious joy, a positive emotion, or having an orgasm, even can be caused by taking some drugs or medication. Chemical induced euphoria has side effects and is generally not favorable for the subject. Unjustified or drug-induced euphoria such as antidepressants, may or may not be a characteristic symptom of a manic or hypomanic episode in people who have bipolar disorder, a psychiatric disorder encompassed within mood disorders.

Modulations of Perception

Modulation in the opinion of the time in states induced by psilocybin has been subjectively reported and measured objectively. In such studies, psilocybin significantly reduced in subjects the reproduction of longer time intervals of 2 seconds, affecting their ability to synchronize with ranges higher than two seconds. Recent studies on the effects of psilocybin on the reproduction of time intervals may shed light on the qualitative alterations of the perception of time in experimentally induced altered states of consciousness, mystical states and psychopathology.

This modulation of the perception of time makes the subjects perceive the present moment as eternity, questioning the pre-established concepts of time of certain modern industrial societies.

How to Avoid a Negative Experience

The term "bad trip" describes a reaction accompanied by varying degrees of anxiety, unpleasant feelings or sometimes unreasonable behavior. The name is generally applied when describing a result that is characterized primarily by panic or other unpleasant sensations as the most memorable part of the psychedelic experience.

Psilocybin opens the mind for broader experiences and leaves the individual more susceptible to external energy. The tense and negative social environment can serve as a factor that causes the feeling of panic. To avoid the negative experience, one must be mentally ready and prepare a comfortable and safe environment, without excessive noise or energy sources.

Possible Adverse Psychiatric Effects

Panic reactions can develop after the consumption of fungi containing psilocybin, especially if ingestion is accidental or happens in some unexpected way. For example, results such as violence, aggression, homicidal or suicidal attempts, schizoid psychosis prolonged, and convulsions have been reported in some publications.

The similarity of psilocybin-induced symptoms with those of schizophrenia has led to the drug being used in behavioral or neuroimaging studies of this disorder. In both cases, psychotic symptoms are thought to arise from a "poor activation of sensory also cognitive information" in the brain that eventually lead to "cognitive fragmentation and psychosis".

What about Addiction?

The Set & Setting

Set and Setting describes the context of psychoactive and particularly psychedelic experiences:

The mentality (shortened to "establish") and the physical and social environment (the environment) in which the user has encountered.

This is particularly important for psychedelic events in a therapeutic or recreational setting. The expression was invented by Norman Zinberg and was publicly affirmed by researchers under psychedelic therapy.

"Set" is the mental state that a person brings to the experience, such as thoughts, moods and expectations.

"Environment" is the physical and social environment. Social support networks have proven to be particularly crucial in the outcome of the psychedelic experience. They can control or guide the course of the experience, both consciously and unconsciously. Stress, fear, or an unpleasant environment can result in an unpleasant experience (bad trip). On the contrary, a relaxed and curious person in a temperate, warm and secure situation is more prone to have a pleasing activity.

Yes, the drug dose does not deliver the transcending experience. It only serves as a synthetic solution: it opens the mind, releases the nervous system from its habitual patterns and arrangements. The view of the occurrence depends almost entirely on the environment. The mechanism of the person, including his character building and his mood at the moment, is critical.

Manuals or guides are necessary. Its goal is to provide a person to get the new realities of increased awareness, to work as a way for new interior territories that modern science has made accessible.

In 1966, Timothy Leary handled a set of tests including dimethyltryptamine (DMT) with controlled regulation and adjustment. The objective was to see if the DMT, which at that time had been considered mostly as a terror-inducing drug, could create delightful activities under a whole and supportive surroundings. The goal was achieved due to controlled Set & Setting.

The "Set"

It is one of the fundamental factors that affect the effect of drugs on an individual. It's about your beliefs, attitudes, knowledge and other thoughts. A clear example of the significant influence that the Set has is the phenomenon of the placebo effect. In that case, a substance that has no pharmacological property can still generate a physiological response as if it had it, only by the beliefs and thoughts (the Set) of the person.

Another important factor within the Set is a person's expectations regarding a drug. These expectations may come from several places, experiences that you have had directly with the medicine for having consumed it previously or indirect skills such as the media, the social circle, etc. The expectations of what one thinks the drug is going to do affect the effects it has beyond its pharmacological action.

The deterioration in a motor task under the influence of alcohol was less for experienced drinkers. They expected moderate damage to the job even when they were told that it would severely affect their performance. Something similar was observed about marijuana users. Those who expected a feeling of relaxation were more likely to experience that. Those subjects who expected effects of anxiety and "loss of control" suffered those effects.

This happens with many other drugs besides alcohol and marijuana. It is also related to how the user interprets the specific effects of the substance. Some may understand the same impact positively or negatively, which affects the experience. In summary, a good Set is a crucial aspect to keep in mind to have a positive experience with a particular substance. It looks like what we think is going to happen, and predisposes us to the experience we are going to have. To have a good "Set", it is essential to inform yourself very well about the drug to be taken, to contrast and comparing results and opinions from trusted sites.

What Is the Setting?

It is the other non-pharmacological determining factor in the experience of a drug. It refers to the environment in which the individual consumes the drug. This environment involves a wide range of issues from the laws and government policies on a particular substance to the immediate environment where a drug is consumed. The latter includes the physical place as well as the people who are in it. An example of the impact of Setting is the difference in the effects that alcohol produces in different situations. On the one hand, when consumed socially and on the other when consumed while alone.

The Setting

It is an aspect that affects the experience of many drugs, and the effect varies according to the environment. From an environment that fosters certain positive moods, where a person feels safe, with music that is of personal pleasure or people with whom they have confidence, to an environment that fosters negative feelings, with people that the user does not know. He doesn't feel safe, or with people, he doesn't trust and thinks he's being judged.

Because They Are Important?

The Set & Setting are two factors that affect the experience with all substances significantly. This varies to a different degree, depending on the type of content and other factors. Some drugs are more susceptible to the effects that Set & Setting have, such as LSD. Even so, these two aspects should always be taken into account when consuming any substance. A bad Set & Setting can trigger a very traumatic experience with a material. On the contrary, a suitable Set & Setting usually guarantees positive experiences with any drug. The great importance of these two factors in influencing the user experience is then seen.

In summary, the Set refers to the emotional state of the individual at the time of consumption. The Setting refers to the environment in which the individual is. This also implies how the user feels about this environment.

Addiction and Toxicity

First of all, it is essential to take into account a point on which all documents, even those reluctant to use psychoactive fungi, have in common. We mean that fungi that contain psilocybin or psilocin do not cause addiction. This is considered to be so on both a physical and psychic level. Concerning physical dependence, which is usually caused by the habituation of the organism to a substance whose subsequent lack produces a withdrawal syndrome, the entheogens completely lack this phenomenon. In any case, due to the nature of these substances, it isn't straightforward for any addiction to occur, since in repeated administrations during the same day or on consecutive days, the entheogens cease to have effects.

At a psychological level, it is also not likely that the use of entheogens will lead to addiction since the entheogenic experience can be of such great intensity. Or it can reveal such a sophisticated theme that the person who has gone through this experience rarely feels like repeating it without leaving a wide interval of time to integrate or meditate on what happened. As the German philosopher Ernst Jünger commented in an interview with Antonio Escohotado, "Drunkenness is all the more fruitful, spiritually, the more time between the approaches. Once a month is better than once a week, and once a year better than once a month".

At the toxicity level, psilocybin mushrooms are considered to be of low toxicity (the case of Amanita muscaria should be treated separately, as it does not contain the same active ingredients).

Thus, it cannot be assured that psilocybin mushrooms do not lack a risk to physical health since the time of their illegalization no severe studies on the subject have been carried out. But from the observation of the shamans who use these mushrooms regularly - since they are used in their art - and of the western people who have employed them during the last decades. I can deduce more or less specific that these Fungi do not offer an imminent danger to the health of the human organism (this does not mean that the use of psychoactive fungi lacks risk.) Since its main activity is deployed at the psychic level, and it is in this area that it is possible to look for advantages and their risks.

A different perspective that is usually taken into account is to point out the low toxicity of psilocybin and psilocin is its structural similarity with serotonin, a fundamental neurotransmitter that occurs naturally in the human organism. This similarity, which in principle does not ensure the safety of the referred compounds, is generally accepted as a possible indicator to suggest the low toxicity of psilocybin mushrooms.

As for dosages, the case of tryptamines (a group of alkaloids to which psilocybin and psilocin belong) do not have a deadly dose for humans. Accidental ingestion of large amounts of d-lysergic acid diethylamide or psilocybin, which have become several dozen times the usual dose, have not resulted in permanent physiological damage in people who suffered this unexpected trip to the stratosphere of the universe spiritual.

Toxicity of psilocybin is weak; In rats, the average lethal dose (LD 50) is approximately 280 mg/kg, about one and a half rates higher than that of caffeine. When administered rabbits intravenously, the LD 50 of psilocybin is approximately 12.5 mg/kg. The deadly dose of psilocybin alone is unknown in the case of recreational or medicinal levels and has never been documented; Psilocybin at most corresponds to 1% of the total mushroom weight of *Psilocybe cubensis*, and approximately 1.7 kilograms of dried mushrooms or 17 kilograms of fresh mushrooms would be needed for a 60 kg person to reach the LD 50 of 280 mg/kg measured for the rats.

According to Adam Winstock, a psychiatrist specializing in addictions and founder of the World Drug Survey, "*Hallucinogenic mushrooms are one of the safest drugs in the world*". The most significant risk is making mistakes and ending up eating a poisonous mushroom by mistake.

The World Drug Survey, conducted in 50 countries and with about 120,000 participants, is the most extensive drug study on the planet. Although of the 28,000 people who acknowledged having consumed mushrooms, 81% considered the effects positive, it cannot be said that they are entirely safe.

"Combined with alcohol and in dangerous or unfamiliar spaces increase the risks of accidents, panic, confusion disorientation the fear of losing your mind", said Winstock. Panic attacks and flashbacks are part of the possible adverse effects that users may experience.

To avoid this, Winstock recommends, "plan your experience carefully, in the company of trusted people, in a safe environment and always knowing what type of mushrooms you are consuming".

Although when you consume this type of hallucinogens, the possibility of having a "bad trip" is inevitable, even positive experiences can be extracted from this type of negative experience. In a survey conducted by Roland Griffiths and Robert Jesse in 2016, and for which they interviewed almost 2000 people, 84% of those who said they had received medical treatment during their experience claimed to feel benefited by their experience.

In addition to their recreational use, hallucinogenic mushrooms have proven efficient in treating depression, anxiety and post-traumatic stress.

Psilocybin in Medicine

Psilocybin has been studied as a temporary medication for many diseases. In 1961, Timothy Leary and Richard Alpert carried out the Harvard Psilocybin Project, executing several experiments regarding the intake of psilocybin in the medicine of personality disorders and other purposes in psychological therapies.

A pilot study conducted by Francisco Moreno at the University of Arizona and funded by the Multidisciplinary Association for Psychedelic Studies examined the effects of psilocybin in nine patients with obsessive-compulsive disorder (OCD) He found that psilocybin can be safely administered to patients with OCD resulting in a substantial reduction of symptoms in many of the patients.

Two other studies investigate the possibility that psilocybin can alleviate the psychological suffering associated with cancer. A study, conducted by Charles Grob, involves 12 people with terminal cancer who were given hallucinogen or placebo in two separate sessions. The second study, conducted by Roland Griffiths, administered psilocybin to people who "with a present or past examination of cancer who have the most concern or feel pessimistic about their condition".

Preceding outcomes showed that moderate doses of psilocybin can enhance mood and reduce the anxiety of cases in venerable stages of the disease, and these effects last from two weeks to six months. In 2008, a research team of the Johns Hopkins School of Medicine published guidelines for the responsible management of medical trials with psilocybin and other hallucinogens in humans.

Also, psilocybin has shown promise when it comes to relieving pain caused by cluster headaches, sometimes considered not only as of the most painful of headaches but as "one of the worst illnesses caused by symptoms associated to humanity". During a 2006 study, 22 of 26 group headache cases recorded success in preventing attacks through the use of psilocybin, and 18 of 19 psilocybin users said they had long periods of time without suffering attacks.

Effects of Psilocybin in the Brain

Brain scans of somebody below the control of psilocybin, the active ingredient in certain hallucinogenic mushrooms used in mystical rituals of some cultures, have given scientists the most detailed picture to date of how that experimental drug works and similar ones.

Two parallel investigations have allowed the identification of brain areas where the activity is suppressed by psilocybin. The results of both studies also suggest that this substance helps people experience memories more vividly.

In the first, 30 healthy volunteers were administered psilocybin in their blood, while they were inside magnetic reverberation imaging (MRI) scanners, which measure changes in brain activity. The analyses showed that the activity decreased in regions that act as interconnection centers since they are particularly well connected with other areas.

"Psychedelic substances are seen as drugs that expand the mind, which is why it has been commonly assumed that they work by increasing brain activity. But surprisingly, we have discovered that psilocybin primarily decreases activity in brain areas that have the highest density of connections with other regions", explains Nutt. "We now know that the deactivation of these regions leads to a state in which the environment around us seems odd".

The magnitude of the impacts reported by the members in the experiments, including visions of geometric patterns, unusual bodily sensations and the alteration of the perception of space and time, is correlated with a decrease in blood flow and oxygenation in certain parts of the brain.

The exact functions performed by these areas, the medial prefrontal cortex and the posterior cingulate cortex, are a matter of debate among neurologists. Still, the posterior cingulate cortex is considered to play an essential role in the awareness and perception of one's identity. The medial prefrontal cortex is known to be hyperactive in depression, so the action of psilocybin in this area, cushioning its activity, could be responsible for some of its antidepressant effects in some instances on which there are testimonials.

Psilocybin strengthens memories, making them more vivid.

Also, psilocybin decreased blood flow in the hypothalamus. Blood flow in this region is higher during headaches, which may explain why some patients had claimed to feel a decrease in these symptoms when they were under the effects of psilocybin.

In the second study, ten volunteers read texts that prompted them to think, while they were scanning their brains, in memories associated with strong positive emotions. Participants rated their minds as more vivid after being administered psilocybin, compared to what happened when a placebo was administered. There was also an increase in activity in brain areas that process vision and other sensory information.

The researchers suggest that this could make the substance use as a supplement for some mental therapies in exceptional cases.

"Formal studies have recommended that psilocybin can develop people's mind of emotional well-being and even reduce depression in individuals with anxiety", explains Carhart-Harris. "This is constant with our discovery that psilocybin reduces activity in the medial prefrontal cortex, as do many effective treatments of depression. The effects of psilocybin should continue to be investigated since ours has been only a small study. Still, we are interested in exploring the potential of psilocybin as a therapeutic tool".

1. Are the mushrooms bad for you?

Research paper ranked psilocybin as the safest drug. All medicines can be harmful in certain situations. Different research also shows that magic mushrooms have medications with the lowest rates of emergency room visits after consumption, at least alcohol and alcohol.

2. Psilocybin, an active ingredient in magic mushrooms, is widely used in laboratory research.

The biggest threat to the magical bodies of mushrooms is the poisonous mushroom, which is not the actual psilocybin mushroom.

The question is whether prolonged use, such as weekly microdosing, can have psychological effects, and more information is needed.

Be careful if you choose your mushrooms to avoid poisonous mushrooms. Do your research on how to find truffles.

3. List of side effects or risks affliction:

- "Bad trip" (unpleasant experience)
- Spiritual behavior, from transformation to progress
- The last of the changes in the visualization was "again and again, the dramatic changes in perception, primarily in the visual system, which ranged from one week to one year after use"

- Missing thoughts that lead to dangerous behavior (for example, driving a car)
- "The occurrence of prolonged periods or prolonged psychosis can be prevented or reduced by eliminating people based on past or current trauma or related disorders in primary relationships, such as a biological parent or brother"

You are not advised to take psychedelics, including mushrooms, if you or any of your relatives of the first or second dose in the past or the past have had psychotic disorders, including schizophrenia.

The most common risk, albeit rarely, appears in anxiety, panic, and short-term (within 6 hours) loss of ability to understand the real, long-term, average 3.8 hours. As a rule, they do not need a hospital. Treatment includes supportive treatment and failure for benzodiazepines such as Valium.

4. New users can safely get large doses if they are ready for side effects.

"Non-drug users can safely receive high dose psilocybin in preparation for side effects" - Griffiths et al. 2006.

5. Are there severe dangers from the mushrooms?

Over time there are magic mushrooms that affect the heart and blood pressure. Magic mushrooms have been used by many people, but that does not mean they are guaranteed to be safe. In research laboratories, mushrooms are provided by medical professionals who can offer medicines for high blood pressure.

Magic mushrooms are beneficial medicine and should be treated as such.

6. An overview of common effects:

- The perception of time and space has changed
- It feels like the world is fake
- You feel that you are in a dream (you don't think you are sleeping, everything looks normal, like in a dream)
- The mood changes quickly, sometimes from very good to very negative
- Emotional Behavior
- Embarrassment

- Fatigue (people in CV joints often prefer to lie on the floor or not move too much. This effect seems to be less noticeable with LSD compared to mushrooms).
- Great students
- Hard to resist
- "Minor, temporary increase in blood pressure or heart rate"
- Love
- Anxiety
- Strange ideas
- Noise

"Most of these side effects are severe and take no more than four to six hours while using the medication".

7. Mushrooms have been used for hundreds or thousands of years in Mexico

There were no reported cases of skin disease or illness. This is a great sign!

8. What is the risk of HPPD?

When people turn to HPPD, they often refer to minor visual changes, for example, viewing the curtain and noting that it seems to be moving a bit. Actual testing requirements for HPPD are more complex.

How long is HPPD? The highest competition is 4.1%, as indicated above. The low score is 0.12% (hits two).

"Many members of the 10 US church churches have evaluated our findings, which have taken at least 100 cases over the years or decades, and no one has reported symptoms of HPPD".

"In the end, although millions of doses of hallucinogens have been consumed by humans since the 1960s (SAMHSA, Office of Unsaturated Studies, 2000, 2001), there are only a few reported cases of HPPD".

9. It can reduce the risk of bad trips.

Read about the risks before the transfer

In the session, you will learn to deal with stress or anxiety and brain time

Start with small doses (~ 0.8 g) before larger doses (for example, more than three mushrooms)

10. It is possible that magical mushrooms may not be active.

Research on the use of examples in humans and studies in nonhuman primates has shown that psilocybin has no responsibility or abuse.

Biggest Mistakes

Dosage

The dose is a field to focus on as it covers many factors, including the person's weight. It is not the same if a person weighing 100 kilos takes 1 gram of mushrooms and one of 50 kilos too, because the effects are likely to be more intense in the person of lesser weight. It should be clarified that all the results described below can occur or not, as many depend on each individual and the neurochemistry of each.

The doses, also called rations, can be of different intensities. To make it clearer to understand them, they are separated into 3: Soft, medium and intense.

A soft dose covers the range from 0.25 or 0.30 grams of mushrooms to approximately 0.80 grams. If you are new to this and want to try mushrooms for the first time, not having taken hallucinogens before, it is the best option, as it will allow you to experience a soft and fully controllable sensation, with a relatively short duration and little intense effects. Perfect for making contact with the world of psycho-biblical fungi.

The sensations that can occur most in a mild dose are, and especially at the beginning of the trip are slight nervousness. Slight stomach upset occurs only in some people (due to the digestion of mushrooms (this feeling of nausea usually lasts about 10-15 minutes since it starts to be noticed). Pupil dilation or contraction and involuntary continuous dilation of them caused by the active substance, mild emotional sensitivity also due to the alkaloid; laughter and fun in the environment on some occasions.

The average doses range from 0.80-0.90 grams to 2-2.5gr. I do not recommend a medium dose to someone who wants to make first contact with the mushrooms, but if I consider 1 to 1.3 grams as a ration that can be included within the soft ones, but within these at the top. It is not excessive for someone who has never taken mushrooms, but from 1.5 grams, things change a lot.

With a medium dose the effects that can be felt are generally pupil dilation, visual effects such as effects with starry patterns, auras, much more intense light sensation and positive appreciation of any fire, looking more "intense" and "pretty". You can increase the ability to concentrate or quite the opposite, decrease it, depending on the conditions. An individual, with closed eyes, can experience visual effects such as colour patterns and lights, such as when the eyes are closed very firmly.

In medium-dose trips the increase of thoughts about memories or emotional problems being able to get caught in a thought loop about them or a simple idea or feeling; you can feel ideas about the way of life, gaining a new perspective on the current way of life and behaviour, and being able to change a person's thinking positively; greater empathy and increased emotional sensitivity about feelings of connection with those around you; focus on thoughts about frequently ignored things and give them importance by also gaining feelings of contact with the world and souls of belonging (why am I here?) and thinking about existence gaining positive perspective on it; important sense of time dilation, things happening very slowly.

High doses range from 2.5 grams onwards. There are no cases of an overdose due to the consumption of *Psilocybin cubensis*, since the body itself rejects, through vomiting, excessive consumption (see section "Addiction and Toxicity"). This type of dosage is only recommended for people who have had previous experiences with hallucinogens and want to go up one more level as far as psychedelic effects are concerned. With high doses, new perspectives on the current way of life and behaviour are almost always gained in a much more profound way than with medium doses.

The rise in high-dose trips is usually uncomfortable, mainly because it is a large amount of product and because it is often a much sharper rise. Sometimes the discomfort is not physical but mental associated with feelings of fear and accompanying personal thoughts about the "why I am taking the shot" or "how did I get to this point". The effect of stomach upset and nausea may be higher than in other minor dosages, and may rarely result in vomiting; The uncomfortable effects of the rise generally decrease with familiarity and more excellent knowledge about the safety and nature of the impact of mushrooms. Visualizations with eyes closed are significantly more elaborate and enveloping, with many more patterns of colours and lights.

There may be a spiritual revelation, intense responses to emotions, and loss of ego. Latent psychological crises may surface, the artistic sense can be intensely increased, and there is an intense feeling of asking things, along with a personal connection. A person may think items that don't deserve it are funny or they may laugh inappropriately.

They may feel relaxation and extraordinary entertainment or intense empathy. They become afraid if a bad trip occurs. It can generate extreme temporary dilation, where minute long experiences may seem like they last an extremely long time. The psychonaut will leave the intense journey with ideas and changes of thought that will make him, positively, experience life in a different way.

There are many varieties of *Psilocybe Cubensis* each with its corresponding dosage and potency. Make sure you know exactly what type you are going to consume and what dosage is recommended. This guidance table refers to *Psilocybe Stropharia Cubensis*. Observations: it contains more psilocin than psilocybin, so it will lose potency by keeping it for a long time since psilocin oxidizes quickly. It is the species that is most consumed and sold. Usually, if someone is going to buy mushrooms, they will sell dried *Psilocybes Stropharia Cubensis*.

If we are to discuss about this, we should illustrate the dosage and effect of this product.

Mini macro intake (0.05-0.25 g)

- Meeting training
- Relaxing relaxes and improves body composition
- Physical activity and the joy of daily activities
- Improved endurance exercise
- General increase (leave - no worries or subsequent collapse)
- Free from ongoing symptoms such as depression, anxiety, ADD / ADHD, PTSD
- Mood improvements
- Relieving stress
- Emotional stability
- Attention, existence, peace
- Forget and pity yourself
- More compassion and cooperation
- The fluidity of the conversation
- Improved memory
- Improvements to the route

- Enhanced entertainment through music, art and more
- Improve creativity
- Instinct
- Improve motivation (for example, actively changing your lifestyle)
- Improve focus / productivity
- Increased flow conditions
- Clear and connected thinking
- Improving a positive or negative mood
- Slightly stunning effect

Macro intake (0.25-0.75 g)

- Improve mood, light enjoyment or enjoyment
- Attention, existence, peace
- Forget and pity yourself
- Perspectives
- Free from ongoing symptoms such as depression, anxiety, ADD / ADHD, PTSD

- Improve motivation (for example, actively changing your lifestyle)
- Increased flow conditions
- Clear and connected thinking
- Improvements to the route
- Enhanced entertainment through music, art and more
- Improve creativity
- Instinct
- Meeting training
- Physical activity and the joy of daily activities
- Relaxing relaxes and improves body composition
- Energy efficiency increases
- Long light body
- Improving a positive or negative mood
- Self-initiatives for socialization
- Improved lightweight sensitivity
- Very smooth images, if present
- Possibly the man says

- It's hard to focus and think in the loop
- Problems with some problematic tasks
- Anxiety
- Social problems and discomfort
- Food in the Depression (Too much for comfort, less "entertainment")

Mini intake (0.5-1.5 grams)

- Improve mood, well-being or excitement
- Light to medium-sized images (such as "breathing" environment)
- Sympathy increased
- The fluidity of the conversation
- Self-inspection
- Increased flow conditions
- Improvements to the route
- Enhanced entertainment through music, art and more
- Improve creativity
- Instinct

- Physical activity and the joy of daily activities
- Discover every day exciting and exciting things
- Improved endurance exercise
- Long medium body
- Clear presentation, top or bottom
- Improving a positive or negative mood
- Sound sensory changes
- Extending or shrinking time (slowing down or accelerating)
- Improved lightweight sensitivity
- The likeness of the mannequin
- It's hard to focus and think in the loop
- Some problems at work
- Social problems and discomfort
- Unsafe Diet (lower limbs)

Excessive (2-3.5 g)

- Great joy or pleasure
- Peace
- Mysterious experiences and mysterious emotions
- A change in life that is self-confident or philosophical
- Other ideas flow
- Improve creativity
- Improvements to the route
- Enhanced entertainment through music, art and more
- Discover every day exciting and exciting things
- Solid-body
- Clear presentation, top or bottom
- Emotional transmission, right and wrong
- Opening and closing photos (pattern, juice, etc.)
- Synesthesia

- Extending or shrinking time (slowing down or accelerating)
- Exclusion
- Abnormal physical sensation
- Light Sensitivity
- Student Growth
- Forced barley
- Confusion
- Pervertness
- Fear and Anxiety ("Bad Travel" Experience)
- Difficulties in the intellectual process
- Poisoning
- Like it

Overdose (5+ g)

- Great joy or pleasure
- Mysterious experiences and intense emotions

- A change in life that is self-confident or philosophical
- The death of the Ego
- Other ideas flow
- Improve creativity
- Improvements to the route
- Discover every day exciting and exciting things
- Clear presentation, top, bottom
- Emotional transmission, right and wrong
- Excellent eye-opening and closing (for example, memories come to life)
- Visual, Audioreal, and design firm
- Synesthesia
- Time to waste
- Thinking Posh
- Exclusion
- Abnormal physical sensations and changes in perception of well-being
- Light Sensitivity
- Great student outreach

- Forced barley
- Confusion
- Pervert
- Invalid engine features (recommended by the nurse!)
- Serious tucks

Effects of Magic Mushrooms

Good Roll

- Laughter and some euphoria are typical of the early stages of the trip or with the use of low doses.

- Subsequently, the user usually goes into a state of calm and tranquillity, accompanied by a marked sense of transparency and mental clarity, so marked that it is common that the new perspective from which things are seen is interpreted as a real revelation. Such revelations may refer to each person's scope or to metaphysical or religious issues that concern all of humanity or the entire universe.

- The perception of the world is disrupted: time slows down, the notion of past, present and future is directly accelerated or disappeared. The colours shine differently, the shapes are deformed, strange lights or sounds and visions are perceived with the eyes closed, until, with the use of high doses, you even see more with the eyes closed than open ("close your eyes, and you will see").

- All this can be lived as something fascinating, overwhelming mind, stunning and beautiful, and this can lead us to an emotional state of authentic satisfaction and gratification, a state that will often be shared with the rest of the people present, being able to establish communication and emotional ties that are unusually intense.

Bad Roll

- However, the alteration of emotions, perceptions and thinking, will not always present a kind and funny face. What is perceived can entirely be lived as horrifying and distressing.

- The change of perspective in a way of thinking might well lead us to say something like: "I don't understand anything about this world". Mystical revelations could lead us to visit Hell instead of Heaven, just as metaphysical revelations could make us understand that not only are we are miserable, but so is all of humanity.

- In short, laughter could turn into tears and calm into panic and anxiety. It is not uncommon for the same trip to pass successively through both pleasant and distressing moments.

- Any change in the environment, in what we do or in what comes to mind, can redirect the experience in one way or another and make us go from fascination to horror or vice versa. For this reason, in the face of unpleasant sensations, one has the opportunity to redirect the trip to something more pleasant by merely trying to think about other things, do something different or change the environment (music, site, etc.).

- However, sometimes (especially with high doses) this can be very difficult, and the person can be caught in a kind of vicious circle with recurring thoughts on the same subject ("I have gone crazy" or "they are persecuting me") who is unable to get out of his head. This is a "BAD TRIP".

- Some believe that even a bad trip can be understood from a positive point of view since they affirm that from bad experiences, one can learn as much or more than from good ones. Moreover, there is less doubt that he is having a bad time and taking the positive side may not be so simple: it requires work, self-analysis and reflection (perhaps that is why many people do not want to hear or talk about bad trips).

The "Bad Trip"

How to make a wrong journey

If someone is having a bad trip, we must try to get the person (as if it were the case) to relax and calm down.

Please do not leave the person alone.

Never try to reassure him with slaps or another violent behaviour.

Don't whisper with other people in your presence or it could increase your paranoia.

If you intend to reassure someone, you must appear calm: no shouting, fuss or nervousness.

If you are in a noisy or crowded place, you should take the person to a less busy place.

You should talk slowly and respect the person's willingness to speak or keep silent.

You shouldn't force the person to speak or listen to you. You should tell them to breathe slowly and deeply, and if necessary, you should set the pace for them.

You should remind them they have consumed mushrooms and are having a bad trip that will diminish as the effects go away.

This may be enough for relatively mild bad trips.

Sometimes, however, the person will be impervious to any objective approach you propose ("it is because of the mushrooms, it will happen to you"), so it will be convenient to limit yourself to transmitting a sense of security: A hand on the shoulder, a jacket or a blanket that covers him, eyes closed, slow breathing, quiet music and only small phrases of support such as "let yourself be carried away by experience" or "move on". Because at this point, the only way out of the vicious circle of the bad trip is to give up and let go.

There will also be cases in which the anguish will not cease until the effects of the mushrooms have subsided. Especially then you will have to be patient and stay calm,

If the situation is complicated or the interested party requests it: Call Security!

Legality

A judge acquitted a Mediterranean shopkeeper who sold "bags of smell" because the judge understood that they were NOT for consumption since *Psilocybe Cubensis* mushrooms were inside a bag of machine-sewn cloth, and with a label that said: "Just to be smelled". Several hemp shopkeepers (grow shops) was acquitted despite having psilocybin in their stores, stating that they were mushrooms for their consumption and it was found that they had a small number of fungi.

(Smell Bags. Pedro Caldentey, 2008. Hemp No. 122 February, p. 18)

On the other hand, another judge sentenced Vincent, from the quick shop "Marcha Shop" (Seville) to 4 years in jail, because he sold freshly packed mushrooms with an expiration date. And although his defense lawyer, Mr. Enrique Lerchundi, invoked the official communiqués of the INCB (International Narcotics Control Board) that leave mushrooms, herbs and potions out of international control, it was no use. The judge condemned him based on the article of the Spanish Criminal Code that prohibits in addition to pure substances, "any preparation containing them". And according to the judge, fresh mushrooms vacuum packed with an expiration date were undoubtedly a "preparation".

Psilocybe mushrooms were not included in the list of prohibited drugs, such as Cannabis, coca leaves or Opium Poppy. Still, the author of the legal chapter of the book omits an impressive final paragraph of the INCB report:

"Neither the preparations (for example decoctions for oral consumption) made from plants containing those active ingredients are subject to international control (...) although the INCB recommends that governments consider the possibility of inspecting these materials at the national level if the situation requires it".

It is possible that the arrests so far have been a strict follow-up of the Spanish Government to the recommendations of the INCB, for the moment conclude that international treaties and INCB reports are minimum documents. From there onwards, each country decides whether to repress more, but never less.

Are Spores Legal?

Yes, the spores are legal.

According to Alacannabis's lawyer, regarding spores he wrote in 2005:

"A priori, it would not involve the sale of spores, or bread, any criminal or administrative punishment covered by the Medication Law (...) technically it is possible to sell both spores and fungal bread. All this with the risk of suffering some action of the dull administration. In some cases, the bread was not even intervened, and in others, the people who were intervened have been acquitted".

(Legal Regime of the Hallucinogenic Fungi. Héctor Brotons in the free newspaper "Soft Secrets". December 2005; p. 29).

I hope that these brief notes will help complement Diego de las Casas's nice chapter: "Legal Aspects about Psilocybin Fungi".

The legal situation seems quite confusing. The Spanish Administration, so far, has followed a clear prohibitionist trend. "Psilocybin and psilocin", Eduardo continues, "the psychoactive principles of fungi, are considered drugs for all purposes". Traffic, cultivation, production or promotion of its consumption constitute a crime.

On the other hand, the possession of fresh mushrooms would be legal, while if they are dry, powdered, bagged or encapsulated, it would be penalized. Anyway, it depends a lot on the quantities: a few dried mushrooms could be justified as intended for own consumption, and a large amount of them in the new State would surely be understood as designed for traffic. The same goes for self-cultivation. It all depends on the amounts and the assessment of the judge.

Draws attention to the surprising variety of mushroom consumers that exists. At first sight, it is difficult to think that HR, a conservative-looking thirty-year-old lawyer who prefers to maintain his identity in anonymity, has psychedelic hobbies. Chairing the living room of his house in the bad Madrid neighbourhood of Salamanca, there are four grow-kits of *Stropharia Cubensis*, the most popular of hallucinogenic mushrooms. "I have been fond of fungi for a long time, in general, and hallucinogens, in particular", he says. "The cultivation begins with the spores, which are, as it were, a kind of seed. To get a fungus to be generated, they must be introduced into a soil prepared with organic materials. This process must be carried out under particular conditions of sterility, light, humidity and temperature so that bacteria don't attack it. It is not simple, and preparation is needed. On several occasions, I tried very carefully, but I always failed".

HR takes the issue of self-cultivation seriously: "Fortunately, about seven or eight years ago, a grow-kit began to be sold that includes a plastic pot with the spores already inoculated on the ground. This means that the most complicated part of the process is already done. Also, in the last two years, a new version has appeared with a semi-transparent bag that has an air filter that maintains the humidity conditions. In this more sophisticated model, mushrooms take two or three weeks to begin to leave from the mail, and a minimum of three crops are obtained.

I have managed to get up to seven. The most straightforward *Stropharia Cubensis* kits come from the Netherlands and are purchased online. They cost 50 e and produce 1/4 of a kilo of fresh mushrooms, which dry will be 25 grams and equal dose numbers. I get the feeling that an explosion is coming in the consumption of magic mushrooms". He remained silent for a few seconds before continuing: «I was introduced to this topic by a group of colleagues in their 40s. In their youth, they had been very fond of trips and had moved to mushrooms as who passes from tennis to paddle. Sometimes we organize dinners with this type of mushrooms when cooking as they do not lose their hallucinogenic properties».

International Boom Interestingly, globalization is having its hallucinogenic effects. Magic mushrooms are experiencing a boom in countries like the United Kingdom. A few days ago, The Guardian newspaper commented on the existence of Psyche Deli, a store in the famous Portobello market where they are openly traded. The business owners decided to contact the British Interior Ministry to know precisely what the legal situation was. An officer told them that dried mushrooms, or "altered by man", are considered illegal drugs, but that the cultivation and trade of fresh mushrooms are not prohibited, nor is grow-kits. The people of Psyche Deli immediately contacted producers in the Netherlands.

They estimate that they sell about 50 kilos of mushrooms a week, which is equivalent to 500 individual doses. To avoid problems with the law, they are not promoted as hallucinogens but as decorative elements or intended for mycological research. The groups fighting for the decriminalization of consumption have put their finger on the sore. As Steve Rolls, a spokesman for the Transform agency dedicated to this issue, said, "it is absurd that eating fresh mushrooms is legal, but if they are prepared in an infusion or a tea you can end up with 14 years in jail".

In Japan, the consumption of hallucinogenic mushrooms is also extended, taking advantage of legal gaps. "It's another example of how ridiculous drug legislation can be", continues Steve. Smoking marijuana there can carry a penalty of five years in jail, but there is no penalty for importing, buying or selling magic mushrooms. This happens because they are not classified as narcotics, but as poisonous plants, which means they are legal only if they are not sold for consumption. For this reason, they are offered as decorative elements to beautify Japanese homes.

Mystical trips It is interesting to briefly point out aspects of the ancestral culture associated with magic mushrooms. Dijo, pseudonym of Gabriel González, is a young artist who is dedicated to the development of virtual spaces. He has travelled on numerous occasions to the mountainous region of Oaxaca, in Mexico, where the mythical María Sabina lived.

In that place is Don Patricio, who guides him in his experiences with magic mushrooms. "This is an actual ritual that begins with the trip, and you have to get there, meet people. The whole family participates in mushroom making, from young children to grandparents. For them, it is a process of learning and healing. It is a ceremony that seeks inner knowledge: nothing to do with the idea of taking drugs to escape and have a good time".

The elements for debate are served. "Just before the elections - says Xaquin, from the magazine Hemp - a bill was in progress that aimed to limit the trade of such dangerous plants like thyme or chamomile, and that, of course, included fungi. It is an apparent attempt to leave everything in the hands of large pharmaceutical companies. I get the feeling that, right now, self-cultivation is the most realistic alternative. On the other hand, the network has become the great centre for dissemination and exchange of information on hallucinogenic mushrooms. It is essential to get advice to avoid surprises".

What the Law Says

Legally, psilocybin and psilocin are considered drugs for all purposes.

Trafficking, cultivation, production or facilitation and promotion of its consumption constitute a crime against public health. Mushrooms are considered severely harmful to health, so the sentences for these crimes will go from 3 to 9 years in prison or 9 to 13 years if there are aggravating factors (selling in schools, to minors, etc.) The possession of small amounts destined for self-consumption is not considered a crime but can be punished with fines ranging from 300 to 3,000 Euros.

The property of fresh mushrooms would be legal, and that of dried, powdered, bagged or encapsulated mushrooms would be illegal. However, this also depends on the quantities: a few dried mushrooms could be justified as intended for own consumption, but a large number of fresh mushrooms would surely be understood as designed for traffic.

The possession and sale of spores are not considered a crime, insofar as they do not contain psilocybin or psilocin and therefore cannot be regarded as drugs. Even so, once the spores have given way to the appearance of the fungus, justice will understand that it is a drug.

Printed in Great Britain
by Amazon